WARDING OFF DEMONIC ATTACKS IN JESUS' NAME
Revised & Abridged Edition

Robert Peprah-Gyamfi

THANK YOU JESUS BOOKS

WARDING OFF DEMONIC ATTACKS IN JESUS' NAME
Revised & Abridged Edition

Copyright © 2019 by Robert Peprah-Gyamfi.

All rights reserved.
No part of this book may be reproduced or transmitted in any form or by any means, graphic, electronic, or mechanical, including photocopying, recording, taping or by any information storage or retrieval system, without the permission in writing from the publisher.
Unless otherwise stated, all Scripture quotations are from the King James Version.

THANK YOU JESUS BOOKS
P.O.Box 10649,
Loughborough,
LE11 2FB
UK

www.peprah-gyamfi.com

ISBN: 978-1-916004-67-2

To the Soldier of the Cross battling with the ferocious onslaughts of the enemy; that any demonic attack however fierce or violent will be crushed in Jesus' Name.

No weapon that is formed against thee shall prosper; and every tongue that shall rise against thee in judgment thou shalt condemn. This is the heritage of the servants of the LORD, and their righteousness is of me, saith the LORD.

Isaiah 54:1-2

TABLE OF CONTENTS

ACKNOWLEDGEMENTS	ix
PREFACE	xi
PROLOGUE: YES TO THE SUPERNATURAL; NO TO SUPERSTITION	xv
INTRODUCTION TO THE REVISED AND ABRIDGED EDITION	xvii

PART ONE

1)	TWO BROTHERS TWO DIAMETRICALLY OPPOSED DIRECTIONS	3
2)	MISFORTUNES SELDOM COME ALONE	11
3)	DRAWING INSPIRATION FROM SAUL TURNED PAUL	15
4)	RESORTING TO A PASSION TO HELP FULFIL A BURNING DESIRE	19

PART TWO: REAL TESTIMONY

5)	NEAR COLLAPSE AT THE OUTSKIRTS OF ACCRA	27
6)	THE PHONE CALL THAT KEPT ME GUESSING	33

7)	FACE TO FACE WITH THE ANGEL OF DEATH	35
8)	"FOR WE WRESTLE NOT WITH FLESH AND BLOOD"	43
9)	A SHORT-LIVED RESPITE	47
10)	VALUABLE ADVICE FROM A CONCERNED NURSE	49
11)	MEDICAL CHECK-UP IN GERMANY	55
12)	AN ABRUPT ENDING TO A WEEK'S ASSIGNMENT	61
13)	ONE MOMENT 'MR DOCTOR', THE NEXT 'MR PATIENT'!	65
14)	IN ATTENDANCE AT A MINI UNITED NATIONS GATHERING	73
15)	A GHANAIAN PATIENT UNDER THE CARE OF A NIGERIAN DOCTOR IN THE UK!	75
16)	A DESPERATE ATTEMPT TO APPLY THE BRAKE ON A RACING HEART	81
17)	"GIVE A CLAP OFFERING FOR JESUS!"	85
18)	NEAR SUFFOCATION DEEP UNDER THE SEA BED	89
19)	HEART DISSECTION WITH HIGH-TECH	93
20)	EMBOLDENED FOR BATTLE	97
21)	TO GOD BE THE GLORY	101

22) VICTORY IN THE CROSS OF CALVARY   103

23) THE BATTLE WAGES ON FOR THE
    CHRISTIAN SOLDIER   105

EPILOGUE: WE ARE NOT QUITTERS   107

ACKNOWLEDGEMENTS

My thanks go to the Lord of Heaven and Earth for the good health I continue to enjoy.

Rita, my wife, together with our children Karen, David and Jonathan, also deserve my thanks and appreciation for their support and encouragement, which enabled me to persevere to the successful conclusion of this work

My thanks are also due to Dr Charles Muller of Diadembooks.com for carrying out the editorial work and for writing the preface.

I am indebted, too, to AGES Software for permission to quote the passage by H. Smith. The quotation in question forms part of the CD called *Charles Spurgeons Collection,* Version 2.

PREFACE

I found this work by Dr Peprah-Gyamfi invaluable because of the personal encouragement I have received from it. While it consists of a series of testimonies that show how dependence on God and the power of the Holy Spirit will sustain one throughout one's journey through life, all of the testimonies in effect hang together like a string of pearls, uniting to show how the author overcame obstacles as part of a continuing journey, both to success and health. If we abide in Jesus we can ask for what we need and expect help to overcome obstacles; all we need to do then is "to trust and obey", as the hymn puts it. What this book demonstrates is that the instances of God's help we receive in our lives are not isolated instances of divine intervention; instead, they constitute a journey that reveals His ongoing love and power in our lives as we grow in spirit and faith, learning as we grow to rely more on Him, and to find our security more and more in his love and his Word. Thus the author, as a soldier of Christ, reveals in his book a journey of faith, and a journey of dependence as he encounters the resistance of the powers of darkness—a resistance that tightens in proportion to his growth of faith!

It is this journey of faith that is very evident especially in the earlier pages of the book, for the author had to overcome his own doubts in the face of evidence that his ministry as a Christian author was increasingly causing him to become financially impoverished. Like the Apostle Paul who earned his funds as a tentmaker to finance his ministry, Dr Peprah-Gyamfi chose a medical career to finance his service as a soldier and disciple of Christ. He might have chosen to become a pastor, which is an honourable and blessed calling, but instead he chose in a sense the steeper route up the summit of his mission. Accordingly, the obstacles placed in his way were all the more challenging. At times he might have faltered, and might have been close to doing so, but he prevailed. He qualified first as a medical doctor in Germany under very difficult circumstances; then proceeded to England where he continued to practise as a doctor, most recently as a prison doctor, but ultimately all for the sake of continuing to write and publish books that proclaim the saving power and grace of our spiritual Doctor Jesus who heals through the miraculous power of the resurrection. In the face of growing atheism, especially as manifested in the work of Richard Dawkins, our doctor-author had no choice but to speak out and produce a book that showed that the human body is so miraculously and wonderfully put together that only a divine Creator could have designed it. What the early pages of the book now in your hands shows is a journey of faith, for our author never gave up and was relentlessly driven forward by his calling.

It all paid dividends, of course, for in the end he was led to find the most rewarding market for his books in his home country of Ghana. But, even so, the success that followed this quickly attracted the attention of the enemy who marshalled his forces of darkness, his principalities and powers, to throttle and silence this upstart solder of Christ for good by an onslaught on his heart, that marvellously designed pumping mechanism that had kept him alive for over half a century! The need to overcome this onslaught has resulted in the series of testimonies that make up most of this book, which again reveal a battle in progress and a final victory of faith and conquest. They all illustrate that wonderful statement by the Apostle Paul that "in all things God works for the good of those who love him, who have been called according to his purpose" (Romans 8:28. NIV).

Those who have climbed the mountain of faith and learnt to trust and obey our commander, our Lord and King, as Dr Peprah-Gyamfi has learnt to do, will likewise achieve the final victory against the attacks of the enemy, for we have our great commander's assurance of victory in His word—especially as expressed in Psalm 121: 1-2 (Good News Bible):

I look to the mountains; where will my help come from? Our help comes from the Lord who made heaven and earth, who will not let you fall for he is our protector who is always awake.

Charles Muller
MA (Wales), PhD (London), DLitt (UFS), DEd (SA)
Diadem Books

PROLOGUE

YES TO THE SUPERNATURAL; NO TO SUPERSTITION

I want to make one thing clear from the outset: please do not count me among the superstitious, among those who hold to beliefs or notions that particular events could bring good or bad luck. For example, there are those who associate the number 13 with bad luck. On account of this there are several places in the world where the number 13 is skipped when it comes to numbering rooms of guest houses, hotels, hospitals, etc. In the same vein, many hold on to the notion that if the 13th day of the month is Friday, it is an unlucky day. Some also hold to the belief that a black cat crossing one's path denotes bad luck or misfortune.

There are indeed many superstitious beliefs around. You may, dear reader, be familiar with some of them. No, I am not superstitious. I must admit that I used to hold superstitious beliefs, but I discarded such beliefs from the very day I decided to follow the Lord Jesus Christ, the Prince of Peace and Lord of Lords, He who was, is and evermore shall be.

The fact that I do not hold superstitious beliefs does not, however, imply that I do not believe in the supernatural. In the same way that I do not want to be counted among the superstitious, I also do not want to be counted among those who, mainly or partly as a result of the insight they have gained in scientific research, deny the existence of anything that cannot be verified through the lens of scientific research. Indeed, such individuals repudiate the supernatural realm of our existence. Though there are innumerable references in the Bible pointing to the existence of Almighty God, individuals belonging to this group hold tenaciously to their views.

Yes, I am a Christian; I do believe in Almighty God, the Power that created the universe and all that it entails. Believing in Almighty God inevitable leads me to believe in the existence of Satan and his demonic host that is made up of principalities, wizards, witchcraft, voodoos, etc.

The Bible states in Ephesians 6:12: *For we wrestle not against flesh and blood, but against principalities, against powers, against the rulers of the darkness of this world, against spiritual wickedness in high places.*

Yes, without doubt, much as I do believe in Almighty God, I also do not deny the existence of principalities, powers, spiritual wickedness in high places bent on destroying and annihilating us.

In the fierce spiritual battle ranging between the forces of Light and darkness, whoever sides with Almighty God inevitably finds himself in opposition to the Devil and the demonic hosts bent on destroying the children of God.

In Psalm 91: 1-2 we read:

> *He that dwelleth in the secret place of the most High*
> *shall abide under the shadow of the Almighty.*
> *I will say of the LORD, He is my refuge and my fortress:*
> *my God; in him will I trust.*

Indeed, left to us alone, we are helpless before the principalities and powers of darkness bent on destroying us. As long as the child of God dwells *in the secret place of the most High* he/she does not have to fear Satan and his demonic hosts, for surely *"greater is he that is in you, than he that is in the world."* (1 John 4:4)

INTRODUCTION TO THE REVISED AND ABRIDGED EDITION

On a visit to my native Ghana in 2011, I experienced weird symptoms which were initially felt in the head and moments later affected the heart as well.

Over the next several months, the symptoms kept recurring. After undergoing extensive medical checks in Germany, an organic cause was excluded. Put another way, the test failed to establish any physical changes in my body to explain the symptoms.

That led me to suspect I could be a victim of attack by the principalities and powers referred to in Ephesians 6:12: *For we wrestle not against flesh and blood, but against principalities, against powers, against the rulers of the darkness of this world, against spiritual wickedness in high places.*

I published my experience in a book, which I titled *Warding off Demonic Attacks In Jesus' Name: Amazing Testimony of Divine Intervention in our time.* In my book I did not specifically point accusing fingers at anyone. I presumed however that it could be due to a couple of local book sellers I had met at an event in Kumasi, Ghana's second largest city. My suspicion was based on the fact that they gave me and my team the cold shoulder when they realised we might encroach on their terrain and in so doing, slice away part of the cake they had until then been enjoying alone. Had they possibly resorted to juju to eliminate me from the scene?

A series of mishaps, adversities, setbacks, etc., that have visited me since I published the original edition of this book has in the meantime led me to change my mind. In considering the catalogue of misfortunes that have been my lot over the years, I recently cried out in exasperation to myself: "My God, what on earth is going on in my life!"

A Twi saying has it that *aboa bi beka wo a na, ofiri wo ntoma mu*. It is not easy to translate it word for word into English so I will only attempt an approximate reproduction. The adage, yes maxim, is saying that if one wants to find out the source of an insect bite on the body, one is advised to search the clothing one is wearing before looking for an outside source. One could also put it this way—your closest acquaintance may well be your chief adversary.

Yet another saying has it that one does not have to wash one's dirty linen in public. In other words, we are admonished not to talk about our private family problems in public.

Even though several factors I am about to touch on have led me to, as it were, suspect "enemies within" to be behind my woes, I have in keeping with the above saying admonishing us not to talk about family issues in public, over the years wrestled with myself as to whether it is wise to go public with my thoughts and suspicions.

Despite my initial reservations, I have finally decided to make my thoughts or suspicions known. In my view, a factor I will touch upon shortly should override my considerations, even if it places a strain on family harmony.

I shall explain the matter further.

Since my arrival in the Western world several years ago, I have observed with bewilderment the mindset of a good proportion of the population that is geared towards the rejection of the existence of anything that is not scientifically proven. For this group of people, anything that is not scientifically proven should be cast into the dustbin.

This type of worldview has led to two unfortunate developments in such societies—the spread of atheism and the marginalisation of Christianity.

If indeed everything, including the way the universe and life in it came into being can be explained by science, then we might well ask what is the need to believe in God?

As my own little way of challenging this worldview, I have decided to narrate the experiences that I and other members of my extended family have had over the years, experiences that in my view cannot be explained away rationally, indeed experiences that blend the physical with the spiritual, the seen with the unseen world.

Having said that by way of general introduction, I want to take the reader through a short excursion—by way of a story of two brothers who despite being very close at the beginning, develop in two diametrically opposed directions.

PART ONE

-1-

TWO BROTHERS TWO DIAMETRICALLY OPPOSED DIRECTIONS

I WAS BORN in a little village called Mpintimpi. The little settlement is situated about 150km to the north-west of Accra, Ghana's capital. Mother had eight children with Father. I had four senior brothers and three junior sisters. As I write today in February 2019, two of my seven siblings, my most senior brother Emmanuel and Sarah my sister who came directly after me in the family ladder, are no longer alive.

After he had been married to Mother for a little over ten years, Father took a second wife. I have six half siblings—children of my stepmother.

My half siblings lived with their mother on a different compound, about three hundred metres from our own.

I developed a close relationship with my brother Kwame, who comes just before me on the family ladder. A few factors accounted for this. In the first place we were only two years apart. Added to this is the fact that as I grew up I quickly caught up with him in height, which caused some strangers to take us for twin brothers.

Mother gave birth to three girls after me. Because of their sex and also the fact that they were younger than myself, they were not ideal playmates for Kwame and me. Our three senior brothers, on their part, seemed more comfortable in the company of their peers than that of their two naughty junior brothers.

Still, other factors contributed to the closeness of Kwame and me during the time we were growing up. The government of the day introduced free and compulsory education just about the time both of us were big enough to attend school. Though several years have elapsed since then I still remember the manner in which the enrolment exercise was carried out for those wishing to begin the academic journey. Each of us was required to use one arm to make a bow over the head and attempt to touch the ear on the other side of his/her body. Whoever was able to do so was deemed mature enough to be enrolled. I managed to do exactly what Kwame managed to accomplish so I was allowed, to my delight, to start school with him.

There was no primary school at Mpintimpi at that time, so both of us, together with other boys and girls of school-going age in the village, had to walk to the next big village, Nyafoman, about two miles to the north to attend the school there.

Although our parents were engaged in traditional African worship, they did not prevent their children from attending church. On several Sundays in the year, Kwame and I could be found seated with other children in the front row of worshippers attending the little Presbyterian church in the village,

The primary school we attended at Nyafoman was run by the Roman Catholic Chruch on behalf of the Ghana Education Service. Consequently, it was known as the Nyafoman Roman Catholic Primary School. The Catholic churches in the area had their district headquarters at Nkawkaw, a large town about twenty-five kilometres to the north of Nyafoman. Occasionally the Catholic "Father" (he happened to be of European descent) travelled from Nkawkaw to visit the local church at Nyafoman. On such occasions, some of the primary school pupils were selected to act as altar or "mass" boys. On not a few occasions, Kwame was assigned such a role.

When I reached Year 5 in primary school an ailment affecting my left ankle (it was later diagnosed as a tuberculosis infection) prevented me from walking the distance to Nyafoman to attend school, a fact that led to a two- year interruption in my education. Though I should have resumed my education two years behind Kwame, I was allowed to jump a year—thus I ended up only a year behind him on the academic ladder.

Our academic pathways diverged even further when, in 1971, I left the village to attend the Oda Secondary School, situated about 70 kilometres to the south of Mpintimpi, as a boarder. Kwame on his part completed his ten-year elementary school education and picked up an appointed as an Elementary School Teacher.

After obtaining my General Certificate of Education (GCE) "O"-Level certificate at the Oda Secondary School in 1976, I was admitted to the Mfantsipim School in Cape Coast, a city situated about 100 kilometres to the west of the capital Accra for my sixth-form. I finished my sixth-form education in June 1978.

In September 1978, at the time when I was awaiting my A-level results, I accepted the invitation of an acquaintance of mine to worship in her church. It was on my first day in the church that I made a conscious decision to follow the Lord Jesus.

Not long after my conversion, I had a dream which showed me on the streets of Europe—a revelation that was fulfilled few years later.

My intention was to study medicine in Ghana. Unfortunately I missed that chance. Another disappointment came when after I had been offered a scholarship to study in the then Soviet Union, my name was dropped from the list of those selected at a later date.

Still determined to realise my goal of becoming a doctor, I left Ghana for Nigeria with the intention of working to earn my ticket for Germany. I had been told that even foreigners did not have to pay for tuition at German universities; I also had an acquaintance who promised to assist me during the initial stages of my stay. After overcoming not a few seemingly insurmountable odds, I finally gained admission to the Hannover Medical School in 1984.

Kwame, on his part, after working as a pupil teacher for a while, decided to engage in farming. In the course of time he met his future wife, a lady from Amantia, mother's home town, situated about 50 kilometres to the south of Mpintimpi. Not long after their meeting they got married to each other.

One day in 1985 an unsettling piece of news which centred around my sister-in-law reached me in Germany: whilst staying with Kwame at Mpintimpi, she suddenly became possessed by a medium, a spirit being (a kind of Voodoo)!

Under the influence of the medium, and to the bewilderment of astonished village residents, she is said to have performed extraordinary deeds and accomplished amazing feats!

In her trance-like state hardly anyone could restrain her; not even the combined efforts of some of the strong men of the settlement could make any influence!

As my late father, who at that time had converted to Christianity and had established a church in the village, later told me, he could just look on in awe as his daughter-in-law began to recount to him some past happenings in his life, of events that took place several years before—events of which no one expected her to have any knowledge!

The news of her possession by the spirits spread like wildfire through the neighbouring villages and soon reached Amantia.

What was to be done? In the end a fetish priest who was already well-established at Amantia was consulted on the matter. The priest revealed that she had been possessed by a deity linked to a river flowing on the outskirts of the village. He advised them to perform a series of rituals—which they duly did. Thus in the next several days and weeks, my sister-in-law underwent one initiation ritual after the other, which culminated in her graduation as a fetish priestess, becoming a junior partner to the already established priest of the little town.

One may well ask what role she plays as a priestess? I have never witnessed her exercising her office. I am merely providing a short summary, based on the information I have obtained from family members at home:

She provides a twice-weekly consultation for her adherents. Her clients seek her assistance on various issues of everyday life, be it medical, social, financial or whatever. From barren women desiring to conceive their own children, to people seeking improvement in their businesses, right down to those afflicted with all kinds of diseases, her devotees consult her hoping for solutions to their problems. The adherents of the religion also go to her to seek protection from witchcraft and juju powers.

The consultation sessions usually begin at dawn and last for a few hours. Shortly before the consultation gets underway the spirit(s) come to possess her. In such a state she is credited with the ability to find solutions to the spiritual, physical and mental needs of her clients.

Clients are not permitted to communicate directly with her. Indeed, the moment the spirits come to possess her, she begins to speak in a strange language—a language that is understood only by a specially trained assistant(s).

Besides the consultation hours just referred to, once every six weeks, she puts up an open display of her powers. The event takes place in a big open arena in the middle of the large fetish compound. To the sound of big African drums, accompanied by rhythmic songs emerging from the throats of dozens of worshippers, she dances powerfully. Occasionally she would fall in a trance. Those possessed by witchcraft, according to the belief of her followers, need to shiver at a moment like that, for it is at such moments, so they believe, that the spirits launch their assault on them.

Was it out of love for his wife? Was it out of personal conviction? Whatever the case, Kwame, instead of holding on to his Christian faith, not only denounced Christianity, but also became an avowed adherent of his wife's religion, even assuming the role of her right-hand man.

Today, he, by his behaviour, creates the impression of being even more entrenched in his wife's fetish religion than she, the possessed, herself!

I am told by my other siblings still resident in Ghana (a few of us are now living outside the country) and other extended family members, that a time came when my sister-in-law actually sought help from a pastor, to request prayers to rid herself of the mediums. Kwame is said to have reacted angrily to that move; in the end he managed to persuade her to maintain the status quo.

On one of my visits to Ghana I visited them at their home in Amantia. As we sat chatting about various issues my attention was drawn to a small, rectangular, roofed, concrete structure built on one corner of the compound.

"What's that for?" I wanted to know.

"That is where we keep images, symbols, replicas, etc., of our deities."

"But I thought it was a single deity?"

"No; initially it was a single deity; she is now possessed by a few more. Do you see the sketch on the wall facing us?" He pointed in the direction.

"Yes."

"That is a depiction of Mami Water,[1] one of our deities."

"When are you going to abandon them for the Lord Jesus, the Son of the Living God!" I asked.

"You worship your God!" he laughed. "We worship our gods! Why do you expect me to abandon my gods for yours!"

"Yours are dead," I smiled. "The Lord Jesus reigns!"

"That is what you believe!" he said, no longer smiling. "Leave me alone to believe in what I believe!"

Those who are not familiar with our culture, especially those who grew up in the West, may want to agree with my brother: "Worship your God and leave me to worship my god(s)! It boils down to the matter of freedom of religious worship!"

If only the matter were as straightforward as that!

In our culture, family members are expected to help each other. The extended family indeed provides a kind of safety net for their members. Such solidarity among family members is particularly important, since there is hardly any state benefit system comparable to the type that prevails in several western societies.

Thus, whether one is at loggerheads with a family member or not; whether one holds diametrically opposite views on matters of religion, politics, philosophy, etc., or not, should such a member find him or herself in difficulty—ill health requiring hospital treatment, inability on his or her part to pay a debt, costs arising from death of the spouse of the individual concerned or even his/her own death—every family member is expected to contribute financially towards meeting the costs arising.

---

[1] Mami Water is a water deity venerated in several parts of West, Central and Southern Africa.

To put it bluntly, in our culture once one is bonded by blood to an individual—however faint the blood relationship goes—one is "till death do us part" bonded, for good or bad.

The fact that I am a doctor currently resident in Europe, also known as *Aburokyire* in Ghana, an area in the world generally regarded by the vast majority of residents at home as a kind of heaven on earth, has raised the expectations of some of my kinsmen and kinswomen beyond the ordinary—and I have over the years done my best to do what is within my means to help other members.

Concerning Kwame, his specific request has been for me to acquire him a mini bus, with which he aims at establishing a commuter business, to transport commuters to and from the next big town about 40 kilometres away. I have so far not been able to meet his demand. Does he feel aggrieved, even neglected by his boyhood mate?

As I have already stated, I have over the last several years been a victim of a catalogue of misfortunes, weird experiences, yes, adverse happenings that have left me baffled, to put it mildly.

I am not pointing a finger of blame at anyone. The question that I put to myself from time to time is—have these misfortunes anything to do with my sister-in-law's mediums?

I am not implying that I am scared by the descent of the agents of Satan right into the midst of our extended family community. In our case, the Enemy has displayed obvious signs of his presence; though he may be invisible in the situations or cases of other sons and daughters of the Living Jesus, his determined attempt to create confusion throughout the world and in particular where God's children are concerned is an established fact.

Indeed, I am not scared by the enemy, for as a Christian I am assured of Divine protection.

That both Kwame and I, indeed very close mates during our childhood, boyhood and adolescent ages, would end up travelling in diametrically opposite directions as far as our religious convictions go, baffles and bewilders me!

In Isaiah 55:8-9(KJV) we read:

> *For my thoughts are not your thoughts, neither are your ways my ways, saith the LORD. For as the heavens are higher than the earth, so are my ways higher than your ways, and my thoughts than your thoughts.*

Has the Lord perhaps a Divine plan for Kwame? As in the case of Saul turned Paul, is He permitting him to walk asunder for a while and meet him in an extraordinary way on "his walk to Damascus"? I can only pray and hope for the best for him.

In the meantime, I want, in the following chapter, to take the reader through only a few of the many mysterious, weird, adverse, untoward happenings or incidents and occurrences affecting not only myself, but also one of my children as well as business.

These indeed are only a selection. I may need to come up with a book to document everything in detail.

-2-

MISFORTUNES SELDOM COME ALONE

THE HEART-WRENCHING CONDITION OF A FAMILY MEMBER

In 1991 I met my future wife Rita in Hannover. We are both members of the Akan population group in Ghana. Our traditional marriage rites required a delegation from my family visiting her family with some presents and performing some customary rites. This family-to-family get-together is obligatory in an Akan marriage ceremony. It is only after such a rite has been performed that the couple can proceed to register their marriage at the registry office and organize a church wedding (or an Islamic marriage ceremony as the case may be).

Rita and I were not in the position to travel to Ghana to be part of the ceremony. I delegated Kwame, the most senior sibling remaining in Ghana at that time and a few other relations to travel to Rita's hometown to perform the rites on my behalf.

Karen, our first child, was born not long after the traditional marriage had been sealed in Ghana. She developed normally. Not so our second child, David, who has been diagnosed with the condition of autism.

On a visit to Ghana in 2007, at the time when David was about 11-years-old, Kwame turned up unannounced at Rita's hometown, having travelled the distance of about 200 kilometres from Mpintimpi. To our surprise he revealed to us that his wife's medium had offered a cure for David's problem! As a first step we would have to sacrifice a sheep. After the sacrificial lamb had been slaughtered he would use part of the blood to smear David's face after which he would perform some additional rituals on his behalf! After undergoing the rituals, he would regain his normal health, he stated. Of course, we categorically declined his offer.

Today, at the age of over 22, David is doubly incontinent for stool and urine.

THE PANICKED GOATS AND THE SOMERSAULTING BUS

In 2011 I visited Ghana to spearhead the campaign to sell my title *Growing Up in A Small African Village* to schools—more of that later. It was during my stay in Ghana that the weird symptoms which affected my brain and heart, which forms the basis for the original edition of this book, happened to me. (More of that later, too.)

I set up a team charged with the distribution of the books to schools using a mini-bus that I purchased. The team was made up of Eyram, the leader; Shadrack, my nephew, the son of my now deceased sister Sarah, as the driver and an assistant.

On one occasion Shadrach drove the bus to the village to visit his mother who was indisposed. During his stay, his mother sent him on an errand to a neighbouring village. He was accompanied by a friend. As they reached the outskirts of the village, all of a sudden a group of goats crossed their path. (It is common practice for residents to allow their domesticated animals to roam about in the village.) In an attempt to prevent a collision, Shadrack applied the brakes sharply, perhaps too sharply. In the event the vehicle was said to have somersaulting several times in the air, coming to rest on its roof a considerable distance away from where it all began.

Miraculously, the occupants, both of whom had failed to fasten their seat belts, escaped completely unscathed! Not the vehicle though, which was badly damaged. Indeed, if it had been in a place like the U.K. it would have been a complete write-off. My team however convinced me it could be repaired. After I had spent a considerable amount on repairs, the mini-bus returned to the road several weeks later, only to be sold for a bargain price a few months later due to persistent breakdowns.

THE CONSUMING FIRE WITH NO ESTABLISHED SOURCE

I had in the meantime acquired a plot of land in Accra, for future development into a cold-storage venture. I erected a makeshift structure on it to serve as a warehouse for my books and also to provide accommodation for the security personnel. To facilitate the delivery of books to schools I had in the meantime acquired yet another mini-van, a VW Transporter. Apart from the security personnel there were a few others staying on the premises.

One Sunday in August 2017 my mobile phone began to ring. On picking it, I was greeted by the voice of Eyram.

"What is the matter?" I inquired after the initial exchange of greetings.

"I have just received a call from an acquaintance of mine, who happened to be driving past your facility. According to him the structure housing the books is on fire! The fire service is at the scene. I am rushing over there to have a look—I just wanted to keep you informed!"

"The warehouse is on fire? Am I hearing you right?"

"That is what I have been told. I am rushing to the scene! I will keep you updated."

"Okay, I am at home, so call as soon as you get there!"

The warehouse on fire! What could have caused it, I wondered?

After about an hour my phone rang again.

"Unfortunately, things do not look good!" Eyram began.

"Go ahead, I'm listening!" I replied in a calm voice. The catalogue of adversities, challenges, difficulties, etc., I have gone though since childhood was making me almost immune to them!

"Unfortunately, the warehouse is completely burnt down!"

"Really?"

"That is not the end of the matter, Doc. The fire was not limited to the structure. Unfortunately, the fire jumped over to the bus which was parked a few metres away. The front side—the driver's area; the bonnet, the engine compartment, have all sustained considerable damage. To put it bluntly—it is burnt beyond repair!"

"What could have caused the fire?" I wanted to know.

"It's a mystery. An electric fault can however be completely excluded. As a result of the *dumsor-dumsor* (erratic power outages) epidemic we are facing in the country, that particular area of the city is experiencing a planned electricity outage. Indeed, as I am speaking to you, electricity is yet to be restored".

"What then could have caused it? Was the security person using his charcoal stove at the time?"

"That can also be ruled out too for he was not around. The only source of the fire could be the few guys who have been granted a temporarily stay there—one of them was asleep and was awakened by the others; the others deny having started any fire!"

Up to today, no specific cause for the fire has been established. Because the wooden structure was only a temporary construction pending the ultimate development of the place, no one had thought of an insurance policy.

Does the reader wish me to continue listing the catalogues of adverse happenings that have visited my home over the last several years? Well, I better reserve the others for a future time, for lack of space and the need to be pertinent without digression from the aim of this particular book project prevents me from further elaboration.

-3-
DRAWING INSPIRATION FROM SAUL TURNED PAUL

HOW DID A MEDICAL DOCTOR currently based in the UK end up travelling down to his native Ghana to market books to schools? The reader deserve an answer to that, for it was during the course of that campaign that the weird symptoms affecting my brain and heart, which form the basis of this narration, first began.

To answer that question, I will take the reader back to my roots, right back to my little village Mpintimpi.

Yes indeed, my desire to study medicine was hatched at the time I was growing up in the little village with the big name!

The human suffering I was exposed to as a child played a not insignificant role to influence my decision. The nearest hospital was located about thirty kilometres away. The population was made up of poor peasants. As a result of the widespread poverty, residents sought medical help at the hospital only as a last resort.

Even if they managed to gather the money needed to pay for their transportation and meet the expected hospital bills, the means of transporting the sick could be a problem, for the road leading from Mpintimpi to Nkawkaw where the hospital is located was less frequented by traffic at that time.

The villagers were small-scale farmers. They grew what they ate and ate what they grew. Accompanying the sick to hospital could cost them a whole day's work on their farms. They could not boast of any government agency that would compensate for the loss.

As a result of the above factors, those who fell ill tended to wait at home and try traditional medicine until their condition deteriorated before seeking conventional medical treatment—in some cases it was too late for them to be helped!

The above and various other adverse factors that negatively influenced the provision of healthcare to the population influenced my decision to study medicine.

Though my parents were poor, I eventually made it all the way to sixth form. At the time I finished my sixth-form education, though I believed in God and attended church sporadically, I could at best be described as a casual Christian.

Just as I was awaiting my A-level result and hoping to enter Ghana medical school, I made a conscious decision to follow the Lord.

Literally on fire for the Lord in the immediate aftermath of my conversion, and burning to work in the service if my new-found love, I was faced with two options—to go straight to Bible School and become a pastor, or first to realise my previously cherished goal of becoming a doctor, after which I would serve the Lord in whichever capacity He found appropriate.

In the end I decided on the second option, for the following reasons:

In the first place I did not want to be a financial burden to the church I would pastor (if any) in the future. Of course I have nothing against a pastor being paid by the church for his/her services. Personally, however, I was fascinated by the example of Apostle Paul who worked as a tentmaker partly to support himself, not wanting to overburden the young churches that he founded.

> *Neither did we eat any man's bread for nought; but wrought with labour and travail night and day, that we might not be chargeable to any of you:*
>
> *Not because we have not power, but to make ourselves an ensample unto you to follow us. For even when we were with you, this we commanded you, that if any would not work, neither should he eat.*
>
> *1 Thessalonians 3:8-10*

So I prayed the Lord to help me to reach medical school, to, as it were, first help me earn a trade, after which I would use my training to further His Kingdom.

I knew the Lord had endowed me with the mental capability to study medicine. What I was lacking was the financial backing. The prevailing educational policy of the country favoured me, though; not only was tuition free up to university level, the state also provided free accommodation and free boarding to students. As if that were not enough, the state also granted students generous loans to be used in the acquisition of textbooks and other educational material.

Things did not go as I had envisaged. In the end I missed the chance to study medicine in Ghana. Next, I tried to obtain a scholarship to study in the then Soviet Union. (At that time countries in the Eastern Bloc annually made available several scholarships for students from the developing world.) That attempt also proved futile.

In the end I left Ghana for Nigeria, with the aim of working to obtain my plane ticket to travel to the then West Germany with the hope of realising my goal of studying medicine. Eventually I gained admission to the Hanover Medical School. (The arduous path I trod from my little village until my admission to the Hanover Medical School in Germany has been laid down in the book *The Call That Changed My Life*.)

-4-

RESORTING TO A PASSION TO HELP FULFIL A BURNING DESIRE

I did not see medicine as an end in itself, but rather as a means to an end. After qualifying as a general practitioner, I began to explore avenues by which I could contribute to the furtherance of the Kingdom of the Alpha and Omega.

One of the things that had been in my heart since my childhood and which had gained prominence after I began studying medicine was to found a hospital in the area I grew up in to provide medical care for the population living there.

How could I come by the money needed for the charity hospital? As I explored all the possible avenues by which I could come by the substantial amount needed, my thoughts went to a capability that I have not yet touched upon—the gift of writing.

I did indeed recognise at a young age the passion not only for reading but also for writing. I made my first attempt to write a book when I was about 14. I had to abandon the project after writing several pages for lack of resources.

My passion for writing followed me to secondary school. Indeed, during my days at my Almar Mater, Oda Secondary School, I contributed on a few occasions to our school magazine.

Just about the time of my conversion, I contributed on a few occasions to the *People's Evening News*, a left of centre newspaper based in Accra, Ghana's capital. In my articles I lashed out at what I perceived as the social and economic inequality prevailing in the country: whereas a minority were living in opulence in the affluent district of Dzorwulu in Accra, the masses were struggling to make ends meet, I moaned.

Despite the little time at my disposal, I pursued my writings while at medical school. On a few occasions my articles were published in two leading German Christian magazines.

So, in this way, I came to draw on the talent just referred to in my bid to realise my goal of setting up a charity hospital.

Though others may consider my expectations overly exaggerated, even blown out of proportion, I dreamt of coming up with a bestseller that could rake in considerable funds, perhaps even millions! Since the money was not meant for my personal use but for the furtherance of the Kingdom of God, something in me urged me to dream big! An internal voice said to me: some indeed dream of earning millions and spending the money in an excursion to planet Mars, so why then not dream of earning millions to enable you build hospitals for the poor and engage in other humanitarian ventures that will have the welfare of groups such as the handicapped, orphans, the homeless, etc., at heart?

The first book idea came to me shortly after graduating from medical school.

One day, as I headed home from my tedious session as a junior doctor at the district hospital in Helmstedt in the German federal state of Lower Saxony, news of the passing away of my mother reached me.

It had all along been my desire to invite Mother, to whom I was closely tied, to Europe to see with her own eyes what we called *Aburokyire* (the land of the European)—the place that conjures up all sorts of fantasies in the minds of the folk at home, the place that many there regard as a kind of heaven on earth, where money, as it were, rains from heaven.

For several reasons, the main being financial, I had continued postponing the invitation. As might be expected, I was very disappointed by the turn of events.

Even more disappointing was the fact that, owing to circumstances beyond my control, I was unable to be at her burial.

As a way of coming to terms with the situation, the idea of the book *A Letter to My Dying Mother: Surviving in the West* was born. In the "letter", delivered by a fictitious courier, I set out to narrate to the gravely ill woman all that she would have experienced had she had the opportunity to visit me in her lifetime.

As with all subsequent books, the book was self-published from my own resources, from part of the earnings from my doctor's work.

Next I wrote *The Call That Changed My Life* which, in a nutshell, is an account of how I made the journey all the way from my little village Mpintimpi to medical school in Germany.

The Call that Changed my Life was followed by *Be Encouraged in Jesus*– verses and poems to encourage and motivate Christians in their daily Christian walk.

In June, 2007, Rita and I took our three children to a journey to Ghana. That was the first time I was visiting my native Ghana in 13 years. Prior to our departure, news had reached us to the effect that the country had undergone quite impressive developments on the economic and political fronts since our last visit.

I was so impressed by the changes I saw that, on our return to the U.K., I decided to write the book *Three Cheers for Ghana*, which apart from describing our own holiday experiences, highlighted the significant developments that had taken place in the country since my last visit in 1994.

Instead of the *millions* I had hoped for from my books to further the Kingdom of God, the book business turned out instead to be a drain on my doctor's income, due to the poor sales which in turn was due to the lack of time on my part to engage in intensive marketing and PR activities.

Still, my passion for writing could not be curtailed.

In 2007 the book *The God Delusion* by Professor Richard Dawkins, a prominent English professor and atheist, hit the bestseller list in many parts of the world. The title created the impression that whoever believed in God had lost his or her mind. That was a notion I could not allow to stand unchallenged. That served as the inspiration for my next title: *Seeing God through the Human Body,* which was published in February 2009. Making reference to the complex build-up of the human body, I stress the fact that the human body is too complicated to have been the result of a chance evolution.

Over a period of six months in 2010, I engaged in a weekly one-hour radio broadcast on an FM Radio Station in London serving mainly the African community there. At the end of the period I decided to publish the sermons under the title *The Christian Soldier's Battle Cry* (July 2010).

The Christian Soldier's Battle Cry was followed by *Dr Jesus, the Doctor who knows no bounds*.

Next I wrote *Growing Up In A Small African Village*, which is an account of how life proceeded in the little village of my birth, Mpintimpi, as I was growing up there. Long before putting the final full stop on my manuscript, I sent excerpts to a few associates of mine in Ghana for further distribution to secondary school head teachers for consideration as reading material in their respective schools.

Just as I was struggling to complete the book, one day I received an e-mail from one of my associates. A pleasant surprise awaited me on reading it: a school in Kumasi, Ghana's second largest city, had pre-ordered 150 copies! In due time the interest in the book spread to various schools in the country, with several of them pre-ordering.

Eventually, the head of the English department of a leading school in the country, who informed me he had recognized the potential of the book to gain widespread acceptance in schools in the country, advised me to print large quantities and set up a marketing team charged with marketing the book to secondary schools nationwide.

Following his advice, I took a substantial loan from a U.K. bank and placed a substantial order with a Chinese printer.

Just as the books were about to be cleared from the port in Ghana, I left the U.K. for Ghana to spearhead the marketing campaign.

I had in the meantime found a personal assistant in the person of Eyram, a young man in his mid-twenties who had just graduated from University. Together with him, I visited various schools in the country to introduce the book to schools.

In the event, word reached us to the effect that the heads of state secondary schools in the Ashanti Region, one of the ten regions of the country, were holding a regional conference in Kumasi, the regional capital.

We decided to attend. As we found out on our arrival, it was not only our team that was looking to take advantage of the meeting—about half a dozen other suppliers were also present.

We interacted with a few of them. In the process, I got the impression the main supplier of English reading books to schools in the region and beyond was not open to competition. Indeed, he made it clear to us that he was the sole supplier of the type of book we were intent on supplying. We should either sell the soft copy to him so he could print copies for further distribution or we should forget ever finding any head teacher in and around the region who would want to order from us. I replied by letting him know that I was open to the idea of selling in bulk to him at a wholesale price subject to negotiation. He in turn could sell to the schools in the region at a profit. My proposal was rejected outright.

Although we did not receive any concrete orders on that occasion, a good number of the heads we met promised to contact us at a later date to place an order.

After spending the night in Kumasi, we left the next day for Mpintimpi.

As might be expected, I was warmly welcomed, not only by members of my family, but by the community at large. The excitement became more intense when they got to know the reason for my stay in Ghana. Almost every resident of the little settlement capable of reading wanted a copy of *Growing Up in a small African village!*

After spending a night at Mpintimpi, we left for Accra the next day.

PART TWO
REAL TESTIMONY

-5-

NEAR COLLAPSE AT THE OUTSKIRTS OF ACCRA

THE JOURNEY to Accra was uneventful. I checked into a hotel on the western outskirts of Accra to spend my few remaining days in Ghana prior to my departure back to the U.K. The hotel served breakfast as part of the accommodation tariff. During the rest of the day, one could eat from their restaurant. The meals were prepared to order. In other words, one could not just go there and order a meal that could be served after a short wait. Instead, one had to place the order several hours ahead of time. As I learnt from the cook, in not a few instances it was after they had received an order that they dispatched some of the kitchen staff to a nearby market to look for the requisite ingredients.

The main cook of the hotel was an elderly man whose age I put at around 70. One evening when he came to serve my dinner, his eyes caught sight of a few copies of *African Village* lying on the writing desk. In doing so he noticed my name on the front cover.

"Did you write that?" he inquired.

"Yes I did. That is the reason I am in the country. I am trying to get the authorities to recommend it for use as a supplementary reader in our schools."

"May I have a copy?"

"Yes of course."

Saying that, I handed him an autographed copy. In the ensuing conversation, he told me something about himself, among others that in the early 60s, at the time of President Nkrumah, then Ghana's president, he used to work at the Peduase Lodge, the presidential holiday resort situated at the top of the Akuapem Ridge, about 40 kilometres to the north-east of Accra.

"That is very interesting. I guess there came a time when you came close to him?"

"Yes indeed."

"Why are you still working," I ventured, adding diplomatically, "at your age?"

"Well, I can do without the meagre income I earn here," he conceded, and explained, "My children have, however, advised me to keep working to keep fit."

On my return from a day's trip to the Central Region to introduce the books to some schools there, I rested in my room for a while before heading for the reception to order one of my favourite local dishes.

The seasoned cook as usual prepared a delicious meal. Though he had on all occasions been generous, he was even more generous on this particular occasion. The meal was so plentiful I decided to enjoy half of it and leave the rest for a later time.

A look at my watch after I had finished eating told me it was 7:30 p.m. local time, which was 8:30 p.m. in the UK. (Ghana is in the GMT or universal time zone. The country usually shares the same time with the United Kingdom; this only changes in summer when the clocks in the United Kingdom are set an hour ahead of GMT.)

Since my arrival in Ghana I had made it a custom to call my family around that time. Thus I began to look out for my mobile phone with the intention of repeating the daily ritual. Just as I got hold of it and attempted to dial our number, the device began to ring! A look on the display revealed where it came from—home!

The conversation with Rita was not out of the ordinary. I told her about our day's trip and the encouraging response from the heads of department we visited. She on her part reported on issues revolving around our children, the unstable U.K. weather and matters of general interest.

I was enjoying the conversation with my other half when I began all of a sudden to experience a peculiar sensation in my head, a feeling difficult to put into words. It was a kind of burning sensation, of the type one experiences in the mouth after eating a hot spicy meal made with chilli pepper.

The burning sensation soon gave way to a kind of hotness, a hotness that engulfed not only the whole of my head, but also spread to the rest of my body. As if that were not enough, shortly after the onset of the weird symptoms I had a feeling as if someone was shaking my heart, like one would swing a pendulum to set it in motion. Moments later my heart felt as if it were jumping to and fro in my chest, as one might on hearing an exciting bit of news. Soon my heart was not only "jumping around", but accelerating, accelerating rapidly, as if in a bid to set a world speed record for the *Guinness Book of World Records*!

The result of the abnormal activities of my heart was that, soon, I began to feel not only dizzy, but very bad indeed. Moments later I was barely able to keep my balance on the chair I was sitting on as the whole world began to spin before my eyes!

Rita was in the middle of narrating an exciting event that had happened during the day. Not wanting her to get a hint of what was happening to me several thousand kilometres away and so as not to cause her distress, I sought an opportunity to end the conversation as quickly as I could.

Happily, she soon ended what she was in the process of narrating. I saw that as an opportunity to end the conversation.

"Okay, let's end it here. I will speak to you about the same time tomorrow. Good night!" I said and placed the phone on the desk.

Meanwhile I felt like collapsing to the floor. With all the strength I could muster I made it to the bed a few metres away. With my whole bodily feeling as if on fire, the world spinning before my eyes and beginning to experience some difficulty breathing, I felt for the first time in my life that I would probably not make it to the next day.

What was I to do? Call the reception for help? What help could they offer apart from an attempt to take me to hospital?

I had since my arrival in the country heard reports concerning an improvement in the health sector. I had learnt that in contrast to the situation that prevailed in the country when I resided there several years ago, there was a quite well-functioning ambulance service. I realised however that getting to hospital from the hotel where I was staying was not going to be easy. The hotel was far removed from the next available hospital. Besides that, the main roads leading from the hotel were terribly congested for the most part of the day. I reckoned it would take several minutes, to get to the Korle Bu hospital, the nearest hospital capable of providing any decent medical assistance.

In the meantime the weird symptoms worsened instead of improving. At that moment I decided to consult the only Doctor available at every time and place, the Greater Physician of our age, the Best Help in time of trouble—yes, the Doctor Who Knows No Bounds, He who is the same yesterday, today and forevermore.

With all the strength left in me I began to pray: "Save me Lord Jesus, save me Lord Jesus; in your mighty Name, save me!" I recited those lines over and over again. I kept doing so for several minutes thereafter.

About half an hour after the onset of the symptoms I began to notice a gradual improvement in my condition. Both the hotness in the head and body reduced in intensity. My heart, while still beating fast, was not going as fast as before.

Finally, about an hour after it all began, I felt strong enough to sit up on the bed.

The Lord is my shepherd, I shall not want; even though I walk through the valley of the shadow of death, I will fear no evil, for though art with me, thy rod and thy staff they comfort me!"

Thus I encouraged myself with these words from Psalm 23.

After sitting for a while, I decided to lie down again. Soon I was overcome by sleep. When I woke up it was a few minutes past midnight. I felt very strong again. As suddenly as I had experienced the burning sensations and giddiness, so had they also vanished!

The able hands of the Living Lord had indeed carried me safely through the valley of the shadow of death. I just could not express my gratitude enough to the Lord for His intervention.

I spent the next several minutes pondering over my experience. The physician that I am, I just could not fathom what could be behind the weird set of symptoms I had just experienced. I had until then enjoyed excellent health. Indeed, I did not remember the last time in more than 25 years that I felt so sick that I had to stay away from lectures or work as the case may be. Throughout my stay in Ghana, I had felt very well. As I drove around with Eyram on that day, I was in very good health, as fit as a fiddle, as it were.

So what was wrong with me? Indeed I was at a loss as to the type of disease or condition that could result in the weird burning sensations to the brain.

What could also be behind the strange behaviour of my heart, indeed, a feeling as if someone was pulling on it to cause it to race out of control?

There are indeed clinical conditions like panic attacks that can all of a sudden cause the heart to race. Imagine, a veteran in the matter of suffering and life challenges suffering a panic attack—and at a time when I was not facing any life situation which could tend to trigger one!

Could it then be from the food—chemical poisoning, perhaps? I wondered how poison in food could lead to a sensation of hotness in the head and brain and the feeling of someone tugging on the heart to cause it to accelerate out of control?!

If food poisoning was indeed the cause of my problem, the question then was—what was the motive of the perpetrator? Or was it a case of accidental poisoning?

Though I had serious doubts that food poisoning could account for the experience of the evening, the fact that I could not find any plausible explanation led me in the end to blame the meal for the strange experience. As a result of that thinking I decided not to eat any further meals from the hotel for the rest of my stay.

For a while I considered reporting the incident to the hotel. After careful thought, however, I decided to abandon the idea. After all, I had no hard evidence to support my case. I also decided not to mention the incident to any other person apart from my family back home in Loughborough, in the U.K.

-6-

THE PHONE CALL THAT KEPT ME GUESSING

My schedule for the next day involved a journey to Akim Oda, a town situated about 100 kilometres to the north-west of Accra. I had planned a visit to Akim Oda Senior High School, my alma mater, to present the school with a few Dell laptops I had brought along from the United Kingdom.

Following the incident of the previous evening, I had during the night considered cancelling the trip. Partly because I did not want to disappoint the school and also due to the fact that I felt well on waking up, I decided to keep to my schedule.

Just as I was about to leave my room for the trip, my mobile phone began to ring. On picking it up I was greeted by the voice of Kwame. It was unexpected! I had met him during my stay at Mpintimpi and presented him with a present I had brought along from Europe.

What had caused him to call me at that time of the day?

"Is everything okay in the village?" I inquired after the initial greetings.

"Yes, indeed."

"Is there anything you want to discuss with me?" I continued.

"Not really. I just called to find out if everything is okay with you."

"Thank God, I am okay," I replied, keeping silent about the experience of the previous evening.

"Good to hear you are fine. Well, as I mentioned just a few minutes ago, I decided to call to check if everything is okay with you. I wish you a nice day."

"Okay, thanks for your concern."

I did not make much out of the conversation at that time; but looking back today, and against the backdrop of the several adverse experiences I have had, some of which the reader is aware of, I begin to ask myself—was it indeed an accidental call?

Just as I reached the reception, Eyram arrived. Together we headed for my former school.

The presentation of the laptops before a special assembly of the whole school went well. Without any incidents, we returned to Accra just before the onset of darkness.

The next day I called on the national chairman of the Conference of the Heads of State Assisted Secondary Schools (CHASS for short) to introduce the book and solicit his help in my effort to spread it to secondary schools in the country. He promised to do all he could to assist. He invited me to attend the impending meeting of the organisation at the beginning of September that year. Almost every head teacher of the over 400 public secondary schools would be attending. It would offer a good opportunity for me to introduce and market the book to them, he said.

I was not unaware of the impending meeting; indeed I was considering attending. Receiving an official invitation to do so by the national chairman strengthened my resolve to attend.

Thus, even as I was preparing to leave Ghana, plans were afoot for my return barely ten weeks later.

I ended my stay in Ghana on Friday July 8 and flew back to the U.K.

As planned, barely seven weeks after my return to the U.K., I headed back to Ghana, on September 2, to attend the said conference. Nothing untoward happened to me during the two-week stay.

-7-

FACE TO FACE WITH THE ANGEL OF DEATH

THE FIRST OPPORTUNITY to earn an income to replenish my depleted coffers following my second stay in Ghana came on Tuesday 20th September. For the next four days till Saturday 24th September, my locum agency had booked me to work full time in one of Her Majesty's Prisons. The prison in question is located south-west of London.

I had been working in the said prison on a part-time basis since October of the previous year. As was my custom, whenever I worked in the said prison I booked into self-catering accommodation on the first day of work. I would stay there till that Saturday.

Thanks to the internet and modern-day communication, I was in contact with my team in Ghana. Schools had reopened and my team had started delivering copies of the book to a few schools.

Though there was an hour's break between the two four-hour sessions I was doing in the prison, I usually stayed on the premises of the prison instead of coming out to, as it were, enjoy the freedom of the outside world.

On the Friday afternoon, however, I decided to make an exception by taking advantage of the break to rush to my accommodation situated about three kilometres away to make an important call to my team in Ghana. Just as I left the main street I was driving on and turned into a smaller street not far from my destination, I was suddenly confronted by a funeral procession. An approximately 50-year-old man who walked ceremoniously in front of the hearse was just a stone's throw from me.

The road was very narrow at that spot, so I had to park my car at the edge of the road to make room for the procession. Almost everyone in the procession, which stretched a considerable distance, was of African descent. Based on the mourning clothes worn by most, I concluded that they were likely from Ghana. I was right, for I soon overheard several of them conversing in *Twi*, which is my mother tongue.

On reaching my accommodation, I quickly made the call and headed back to the prison. On reaching the reception, I overheard the conversation of a staff member who happened to have just arrived for the afternoon duty with another member of staff about a funeral she had just attended.

"This is the first time I have been to a Ghanaian funeral. It was quite remarkable," she said.

At that juncture I approached her. "I bumped into a funeral procession barely an hour ago," I began. I went on to describe the location where it took place.

"Yes, that was precisely the funeral I attended," she replied.

At that juncture she unzipped her handbag and pulled out a picture.

"That is the picture of the deceased," she revealed.

"He looks quite young", I remarked on seeing it.

"Yes, I understand he was in his mid-40s. He was a really lovely individual. One of his children happens to be the classmate of my boy."

"Do you know the cause of death?" I inquired.

"Heart attack; he died suddenly of a heart attack."

"Sad; very sad, indeed!"

"Yes indeed! I understand he left behind three young kids."

As I walked away, I reflected on life—on how it can end suddenly and unexpectedly.

It was a particularly long working day for me—I was booked to work till 10 p.m. I breathed a sigh of relief when I finally got the "marathon duty" behind me. On returning to the guest house, I made my usual daily call to the family. It was a few minutes to midnight when I finally retired to bed. Soon I was overcome by sleep.

The next day, Saturday 24th September, I packed my items from my accommodation, loaded them into the boot of my car and headed for work.

The session on Saturdays began at 10 a.m. and lasted officially till 6 p.m. The actual end of the session depended on the number of prisoners arriving in the establishment on that particular day.

For example, during the riots that began in London and spread to several parts of the country in the summer of 2011, there were instances when the session ended very deep into the night, in some cases not before the early hours of the following day. On the whole, however, the duty doctor could reckon with the end of his/her work for the day around 8 p.m.

Though there are several doctors in the prison weekdays, on Saturdays only one doctor is assigned to work. As the duty doctor, I was expected to visit the unit where inmates with mental health issues are housed as well as a small ward bordering on the said unit where inmates with various medical conditions are admitted until such time that they can be moved to normal locations.

After I had sorted things out at the said locations, I was about to head for the main block to deal with the jobs waiting for me there when one of the male nurses turned to me.

"Doc, I saw you on TV a few days ago!"

"Did you?"

"Yes indeed! I saw you on Love World TV. I found the programme very inspiring."

"Oh, they did show it again then! As a matter of fact, the recording was done in March. I paid them to show it over a seven-day period. Was it because viewers responded well to it? In any case since then they have repeated it on several occasions. During my stay in Ghana in August, someone who had just viewed it, thinking I was in the U.K., sent an SMS to request the price of the book."

"You must be thankful for the publicity."

"Indeed, not only for the free publicity but also for the message they are helping to spread."

"How can one obtain a copy of your book?"

"Which one? I have written several books."

"*The Christian Health Manual.*"

"Unfortunately I do not have a copy with me now. I will take note of that and bring a copy along next time."

As I had expected, a considerable amount of work awaited me on reaching the doctor's room of the main prison building. It consisted in the main of prescription sheets that needed to be rewritten. It took me well over two hours to get the job done. Besides writing and signing prescription sheets, I had to attend to a handful of patients needing urgent medical attention.

I had my lunch break at around 1 p.m. During the weekdays one can eat at the prison canteen. That is not the case during weekends. Usually when I work on Saturdays, I bring some sandwiches and drinks from home. That was not the case on this occasion. To satisfy my hunger and quench my thirst, I headed for the food vending machine at one corner of the large prison. Fortunately I was able to find what I wanted.

About 10 minutes after I had finished my meal I was resting in the doctor's room when suddenly I began to experience a weird feeling of hotness in my brain, similar to that experienced in the hotel in Ghana! But on that occasion I thought it was due to food poisoning. The poison, I argued, could not have followed me to the United Kingdom!

As in the case of my experience in Ghana, the feeling of hotness in the brain soon spread, not only to the whole head but also to the rest of my body! Soon my whole body began to feel as if it were on fire. Was it because of the feeling of hotness in my body? The doctor's room itself appeared hot to me, feeling like an oven.

In prisons the windows are usually small. For security reasons they cannot be fully opened. Instead one can only tilt them. Not only was the window in this particular room small, it could also not be tilted. Instead, one could only turn a knob to allow a small stream of air to flow in, very inadequate in view of the situation I found myself in.

I decided therefore to step outside into a large corridor adjacent to the doctor's room. Not long after I had left the room, I had that feeling, just as in the case of my Ghana experience, of someone taking hold of my heart and shaking it! Soon my heart began to race within me!

Moments later I was feeling dizzy, having to struggle to keep myself steady.

At that stage I decided to return to the doctor's room, to rest on the examination bed. But no, as it turned out, that was no place for relaxation, for the room still felt like an oven to me!

In the meantime I felt short of breath. I decided therefore to leave the building for an open courtyard to enjoy the fresh air outside. When I got outside I spotted a wooden structure—a table and two chairs on each side built as a single block. My heart continued to race within me. Hardly able to stand on my feet, I headed for it and took a seat on one of the chairs. Despite the mild autumn temperatures, my body continued to feel hot. The whole world in the meantime continued spinning before my eyes. I feared I would collapse and fall to the ground at any moment.

During my experience at the hotel, the thought that I could withdraw to the bed offered some consolation; on this occasion, however, there was no such place of respite around me.

The seriousness of my condition had in the meantime come home to me. Without any forewarning, the angel of death seemed to be knocking on my door, seriously threatening to snatch me way!

Did I have time to think about anything at all? Yes, I think I did. Yes, I recall thinking about my two boys, Jonathan and David. It began to dawn on me that I would perhaps not be seeing them anymore, at least not in this life!

I had all along been praying silently to God Almighty to save me. At the point of collapsing, the need for Divine Intervention became even more pressing to me.

"Lord Jesus, help me! Lord Jesus, save me! For the sake of my little children, stretch forth your hand and rescue me!" I cried out in desperation.

I began to look round to ascertain whether there was anyone around whose attention I could draw to my plight. The only fellow humans around happened to be a group of prisoners in an enclosed space about 50 metres from where I was. (Under the supervision of prison officers, prisoners in a small group are allowed into the open from time to time.)

I felt like crying out aloud to draw their attention. But I realised I did not have the strength to cry out.

At this juncture the idea occurred to me to try and return to the main building. There, at least, I could expect help, not least from the nursing staff. How could I walk the approximately 20-metre distance in my situation?

"Help me, Lord! In Your Mighty Name, help me!" I prayed.

Mustering all the strength I could, I got up and began to walk, as I went repeating the line: "In the Name of Jesus, in The Name of Jesus, in the Name of Jesus!"

Soon I was back in the main building. About 15 metres ahead of me, I spotted a nurse who happened to be the lead nurse on duty on that day. With some difficulty I made for her. Initially, she might have thought I was approaching her to talk about a patient or something related to my duty. Soon however she realised all was not well with me.

"What is wrong with you, doc?"

"I need your help, I am not feeling well."

"Come on," she said without delay. "Come and rest in one of the treatment rooms."

Soon we were heading to the said room. In the meantime the news of my condition had spread to two other nurses at work in an adjacent office and both hurried to my aid. After they helped me into a chair, they began to check my vital signs. The blood pressure reading was 87/50mmHG; the heart rate was 155 beats per minute.

For the sake of the layman in such matters, I shall provide a brief interpretation of the results. It is generally held that a normal BP (blood pressure) reading should fall within a range of 110–140 for the top value (known as the systolic pressure) and 60–90 for the lower value (known as the diastolic pressure). The pulse rate at rest is usually between 60 and 80 per minute.

My initial vital signs stated above showed my blood pressure had dropped too low, to a point where it was without doubt of concern. As soon as the machine displayed the reading the lead nurse instructed her subordinates to help me unto a trolley. The trolley was then tilted so I could assume the so-called Trendelenburg position—the head pointing downwards, the legs elevated.

This position has among other things the goal of facilitating blood flow to the brain in patients who for various reasons have experienced a sudden fall in blood pressure.

After the nursing staff had got me in the desired position on the bed, one of them suggested they take my blood sugar reading. I was convinced that was not the cause of my problem; the test belonged to a routine examination under the circumstance so I gave them my approval. It turned out fine.

Just then one of the nurses who had felt my body, began: "Doc, your body feels hot—you seem to have a fever?"

"That is highly unlikely. Indeed, I have felt well throughout the day, until the onset of the symptoms not long ago."

"Still, I want to check your temperature."

It turned out to be normal.

"So what is wrong with you, doc?" the lead nurse wondered.

"I do not know, my dear; I do not know. I have so far been in good health—no heart condition, normal BP, not diabetic. At the time I was coming to work I was fine."

Over the next several minutes the three concerned nurses took good care of me, checking my values at short intervals, preparing a cup of tea for me to, as they put it, "get extra volume into my system", and building me up with encouraging words.

About half an hour after my values were first measured, they began to improve: BP 105/60, pulse 120/min. Not only had they improved, I also began to feel well.

At that stage the lead nurse turned to me and inquired: "Doc, what next? Do you want to leave for home?"

"Well, my home is Loughborough. As you may know, it is about 110 miles [180 kilometres] away! I will rest for a while and decide in the course of the afternoon what to do based on my condition."

"Okay, doc, we will leave you to rest. We shall call on you from time to time to find out if everything is fine."

"Thanks, I am very grateful," I replied.

-8-

"FOR WE WRESTLE NOT WITH FLESH AND BLOOD"

LEFT ALONE, I had time to ponder over what I had gone through. My thoughts went back to the incident in the hotel in Ghana. At that time I had apportioned blame to the food served by the hotel. Now that I had gone through an almost identical experience, it was clear that was not the case. Then there was the nature of the symptoms! How weird were they! Hotness in the brain, hotness in and around the head, hotness in the whole body, the feeling of someone taking hold of my heart and shaking it!

It began to dawn on me, that I could indeed be subjected to an attack by the principalities and powers of darkness.

In our culture, rumours abound concerning the use of supernatural powers—voodoo, juju, witchcraft, wizards, etc.—to influence the course of events in people's lives. Usually such powers are said to be employed by others to adversely affect those they are intended for. They may cause flourishing businesses to collapse, lead to the breakdown of marriages, lead to incurable diseases and even to the untimely death of their victims.

Whereas the influence of such powers may be exaggerated by some, the accounts of their influence are too manifold to be completely brushed aside. I do accept that such accounts may appear strange in the ears of others, especially those in the West.

Whilst in Germany I came into contact with an Austrian lady who spent several years living in Cameroon with her husband, a citizen of that country. She also confessed that prior to her departure for the country she did not believe the accounts of demonic attacks. She admitted that her attitude began to change after living there for a while. According to her, there was an instance when someone whose wife had fallen prey to the advances of another man threatened to eliminate his rival through commanding a lightning strike. And, indeed, it happened—for not long afterwards, the person involved was struck dead by lightning as he rested in his room.

Before becoming a Christian I lived in constant fear of the forces of darkness, of witches, wizards and the principalities. Indeed I harboured a constant fear at the back of my mind that I could become subject to an attack from them. I was a bright pupil, the envy of others, and therefore harboured fears that I could be subject to attacks by the forces of darkness.

All that changed the moment I became a Christian. From that moment onward I was able to rest assured that the "the Lord is my Shepherd" and that therefore "I shall not want".

Yes, I believed in Satan and his demonic hosts; yes, I believed in the principalities and the powers of darkness. Yet I did not fear them, because I was assured that "Greater is He that is in me than he that is in the world"(1 John 4:4). That has been my attitude since I decided to follow the King of Kings and the Lord of Lords.

For the first time since becoming a Christian, however, the awareness sunk deep into me that I was under direct demonic attacks! Of course I had no concrete evidence to support my claim. Nevertheless the circumstantial evidence, as far as I was concerned, was very convincing. Oh, the forces bent on destroying us, my dear Christian friends! Sometimes, I really do wonder! Why cannot the powers bent on destroying us just leave us in peace?

My contemplation was interrupted by the arrival of the lead burse to check on me.

"Is everything okay with you, doc?" she inquired on stepping into the room.

"Thanks for your concern, my dear. Thank God I am still alive!"

After assuring herself that everything was okay with the "patient", she left, promising to come back after a while.

About two hours after it all started I began to feel strong enough to venture onto my feet. I took a few steps around the room. Though still somewhat dizzy, I was quite stable on my feet.

I had three options—to leave for home immediately, to hang around for a while and carry out the essentials, including signing the prescriptions of the new arrivals to the prison to enable them to receive the needed medication and leave for home thereafter, or to stay on till the end of the session. In the end I decided on the second option. Though I did not have the strength to see new patients, I felt strong enough at least to sign prescriptions.

As I mentioned earlier, I was the only doctor around. Failure to carry out my duty would mean the affected inmates would have to forego their medication until Monday. (There is usually no doctor in the prison on Sundays; emergency cases had to be sent to accident and emergency.)

Finally, at about 5:00 p.m., I felt strong enough to set out on the drive home. I could have spent the night with my brother Ransford, who lived just seven miles away. I decided however to drive home. I trusted the Lord who had preserved me earlier in the day to see me safely home.

It was around 8:30 p.m. when I finally reached home. Since that was about the same time I would have arrived at home had I finished the session at 6 p.m., my arrival did not draw any suspicion. In order not to disturb the sleep of any member of the family that night, I decided to wait until the next morning before breaking the news to them. The opportunity to do so came during breakfast.

"So," Rita began on hearing my story, "the food served at the hotel in Ghana is after all not to blame for your previous experience!"

"I must admit I also had my doubts," I agreed. "After all, what would have been the motive? I am really thankful to the Lord that I did not confront the hotel on the matter. No, it was not food poisoning. It was a case of demonic attack; yes, I am subject to demonic attacks!"

"Then you should look inwards, to your own relations, to those who live with mediums!"

"What reason do they have to work against me? After all, I am doing what I can to help everyone," I countered.

"Do you think they are satisfied? They assume you are extremely rich so they are expecting more from you!"

"The traditional extended family in our setting! They all share the same nature! The moment some of the members begin to progress in life, those who feel left behind regard them with envy, jealousy, and even resort to backbiting."

"If only they would leave it at that level! But no, others resort to witchcraft, voodoo, mediums and what have you to try and eliminate such individuals. Once you are out of the way they pounce on your property like hungry lions!"

-9-

A SHORT-LIVED RESPITE

AFTER BREAKFAST I felt strong enough to accompany the family to church. Though some may find it strange, we usually drive a distance of about 90 kilometres to attend church. We started attending the church in question, the Gateway Church near Birmingham, on the recommendation of Rita. She first heard the pastor of the church preaching on Christian Radio. She was so impressed by the simplicity of his powerful preaching that she recommended it to the whole family. I was also impressed when I visited his church for the first time.

The drive to and from church was uneventful. Indeed, for the most part of the day I felt well, as if nothing had happened. That led me to conclude that matters would perhaps take a course similar to the aftermath of the first attack. As it would soon be apparent, that would not be the case.

About three hours after our return from church I was sitting at the dining table enjoying a cup of tea. Rita was getting something done in another corner of the kitchen. We were conversing heartily about issues concerning our relatives at home when, all of a sudden, the now familiar feeling—that of someone pulling on my heart—set in. Following the pattern of previous times, my heart soon began to accelerate; before long I began to feel not only dizzy but short of breath.

Rita, whose back was towards me and becoming aware that I had suddenly stopped contributing to the lively chat, turned to look at me. She noticed all was not well with me.

"What is wrong with you? Has your problem returned?"

"Well, the heart has started racing again!"

A short silence followed. I could only imagine what was going through her mind. That was the first time since we met, almost 20 years to the day, that she saw me in that situation, a situation that was potentially life threatening. How would the family cope should the only breadwinner be incapacitated by disease, and in the worst case scenario called home by He who brought him here?

For the moment, however, I needed to find somewhere to rest, for I felt like collapsing.

"I need to rest for a while," I began and headed for the sofa in the living room.

"Should I call the ambulance?"

"Not yet. I believe all will be well in Jesus' Name."

As I lay on the sofa with the whole world spinning before me, I repeated silently the lines: "In the Name of Jesus I am healed; in the Name of Jesus I am healed; in the name of Jesus I am healed!"

After lying on the sofa for about half an hour, I began to feel better. I felt my pulse; it had in the meantime settled around 100 beats per minute instead of the initial rate of around 140. To ease the anxiety of the rest of the family, I got up and began, as far as I could, to interact with them.

-10-

VALUABLE ADVICE FROM A CONCERNED NURSE

MY AGENCY had booked me to work at the same prison from the Tuesday to the Saturday of the following week, all being full-day assignments. It goes without saying that the family needed the expected earnings badly. As a result I decided not to cancel my engagement but rather do all I could to honour my commitments.

As a self-employed individual, I was bound by the saying: "If you do not go, you do not eat!" Not that I did not have an insurance that would cater for us in case of ill health. In my case, however, the policy kicked in only when the disease condition rendered me permanently incapable of working.

The next day, Monday, my agency called not only to inquire about my health, but also to find out whether I could honour the session scheduled for the following day.

"Yes I can!" was my quick and firm reply.

Doesn't the saying have it that 'Man proposes but God disposes'? The truth entailed in that saying would soon catch up with me. Having felt fine throughout the day, I decided to go to town to get something done. Just as I was about to step in my car to drive back home, the now well-known pattern of symptoms returned with a vengeance. I still needed to drive for about 10 minutes before reaching home. Would I make it or would I collapse on the way home?

> *I will lift up mine eyes unto the hills, from whence cometh my help.*

> *My help cometh from the LORD, which made heaven and earth.*
> *He will not suffer thy foot to be moved: he that keepeth thee will not slumber.*

These words of Psalm 121:1–3 went through my mind as I set out to drive home. As I drove along, my heart still racing, it became clear to me that it was wishful thinking on my part to assume I could honour the session the next day. As I alighted from the vehicle and made it to the door of our home, the words of the lead nurse reverberated through my mind: "Stay at home, doc, and get yourself checked!"

I needed, without further delay, to take steps to get myself checked. Even though the mysterious nature of the attacks led me still to suspect they could be due to demonic attacks, they could well be a manifestation of a disease condition breeding in my body. After all, I could not count myself among the very young of our race. I am past the age of 50 years. My hair, which was deep black in younger years, has in the meantime turned predominantly grey.

I carried my reflections a step further to consider the millions of individuals who arrived in the world about the same time as myself, or even much, much later, who had in the meantime passed away. My being here after all is a privilege, not a right. It could well be that He who sustains me had decided to call me back home. The symptoms I was experiencing could thus be a precedent to an impending Divine call to return home. So it could indeed be that my symptoms had an organic cause—a normal disease condition that had been breeding in my body and that had now begun to manifest itself.

The last time I underwent a thorough medical check was two years earlier. At that time I was visiting Germany with the family. I took advantage of my visit there to have not only myself, but also the rest of the family, checked by my good doctor friend, Joerg. Joerg and his wife, also a doctor, had their GP practice not far from where I used to have mine. At that time everything was fine with all of us. Two years in life, especially when it touches on our health, is a very long time indeed. Anything could have developed in my body during that period.

Having made up my mind concerning the need for a check-up, I was determined to have it done as quickly as possible. As a first step, I called my GP surgery in Loughborough to book an appointment. I told the lady on the phone the reason behind the call and requested an appointment as soon as possible. On hearing what I had to say, she advised me to call the following day. Why could she not give me an appointment that very day, I wondered?

While not wanting to draw a comparison between the UK and German health systems, I had come to cherish the speed at which clinical investigations can be conducted in Germany. I was aware that in Germany most of the necessary tests could be conducted within a matter of days if not on the same day.

With that in mind I decided to travel to Germany for the investigations. Joerg and his wife had in the meantime moved away from Dusseldorf, though not so my good friend Michael. He used to be my direct neighbour in our home in Kaarst, a small town to the north of Dusseldorf. At that time he was engaged in postgraduate training to become a specialist physician. He had in the meantime qualified in that field of medicine and set up his own practice in the city that happens to be the capital of the German state of North Rhine Westphalia.

I decided to call him without delay to explain my situation and request an urgent appointment.

"No problem, you can come a day after tomorrow if you can," he said on hearing my story. "We are open from 8:00 a.m. I advise that you come as early as you can. Do not eat before coming. We shall do blood tests and ECG [electrocardiogram], both at rest and under exercise."

"Can you do echo [echocardiography] as well?"

"You let us do the ECG first. If need be, I will refer you to a cardiologist for the echo."

"Thank you so much for your help. I will be there first thing on Wednesday."

I began to ponder on life, yes, on how unpredictable it could be. Indeed, if anyone had told me a week before that I would be heading for Germany for urgent medical tests, I would have laughed in his or her face!

Since moving to the United Kingdom from Germany in 2006, I had on several occasions returned for a visit. I had on all occasions travelled by road, driving my own vehicle. On this occasion, however, I decided to go by air.

Soon I was sitting behind my computer looking for the next available flight to Dusseldorf the next day. Eventually I found a Lufthansa flight from Birmingham, which is about 70 kilometres to the south-west of Loughborough. When I called out the price for the flight, Karen, who on several occasions had flown with the same flight to Dusseldorf, could only shake her head, for the cost was almost double what she had been paying. The reason was not difficult to find. She usually booked the flight weeks ahead of schedule. In my case with barely 24 hours to go before the flight with probably only a few seats left, the mechanisms of the market had forced the price up.

That was however not the time to occupy my mind with the mechanisms of the free market. What was important for me was to get the means to arrive at my destination quickly and safely, have the necessary tests carried out and put the uncertainty behind me. If I were gravely ill, I needed to know that as soon as possible to enable me sort out my life before the final whistle went for me to pack my bags and depart the transit hall of life.

I left home in good time the next day for the approximately one hour's drive to Birmingham Airport. As I drove along, my prayer was that the Lord would preserve me from any possible attacks during the little over an hour's flight. I have heard and read about instances where there have been medical emergencies during flights, in some instances when the plane happened to be tens of thousands of metres above the earth's surface.

"If there is any doctor on board, would you please come forward; your urgent assistance is required." That is the announcement those who have witnessed such dramatic moments say usually issues from the loudspeaker system of the man-made bird. A doctor I once came in contact with told of his experience during a flight. According to him, he was relaxing in his seat, already rejoicing at the thought of the impending reunion with his family, when an announcement similar to the above was made. It turned out that one of the patients with a heart condition had begun to experience chest pains. He responded to the call and headed for the patient, an elderly man in his 70s. According to him, though he did not have to do anything beyond the ordinary, his presence alone seemed to have been enough to calm the patient until they made an emergency landing at the next available airport. Several days later he received a letter of thanks from the airline involved.

Whenever I board a plane, my prayer to the Lord is to preserve me from a similar situation. Not that I do not possess enough self-confidence to face such a situation. I am a doctor, not a master of every imaginable disease. What if I were to be confronted with a condition that is beyond my professional competence? The thought that I could myself trigger an emergency situation far above the skies that could force an emergency landing far away from home and also my intended destination was unnerving, to say the least.

Happily, the flight was uneventful. We touched down on schedule at a few minutes past 10 p.m. local time. Kofi, a cousin of Rita's, was at the airport to meet me. I had called him the previous day to inform him of my arrival, and he had agreed to play host to me.

In order not to cause our respective extended family members any distress, we had decided to keep them in the dark pending the outcome of the investigations. In the case of my host, I only told him I was there for a short medical check-up.

-11-
MEDICAL CHECK-UP IN GERMANY

I LEFT KOFI'S HOME shortly after 7.00 a.m. the next morning and headed for Michael's practice. Coincidentally, my host's apartment, as it happened, was not far from the practice.

On my arrival I had hardly taken off my coat and taken my seat in the waiting room when a nurse, smiling broadly, approached me.

"Doc, please follow me."

I was led to one of the several cubicles.

"We shall soon take a sample of your blood. In the meantime may I ask you to provide us with a urine sample?"

So saying, she handed me a small container and directed me to the toilet. Moments later I was back in my seat, having done what was requested of me.

Next was the taking of the blood sample. Soon that was also behind me. Moments after the blood sample had been taken another assistant came to request me to follow her.

"I have been asked to do the ECG," she said. "Please remove the clothes from the upper part of your body and get onto the examination bed."

For those not familiar with the term I will provide a brief explanation: ECG (electrocardiogram) is a test that measures the electrical activity of the heart. It allows problems with the heart's rhythm and the conduction of impulses brought about by disease to be identified.

No sooner had I taken my place on the bed than she went about to stick the ECG electrodes to my body. The last time I had taken the test was several years before. It was done as part of a routine check prior to my being signed on as a junior doctor. At that time, apart from what is known as 'an incomplete right bundle branch block', everything was fine.

For the sake of the layman in such matters, I shall pause to give a short explanation of the term. 'Bundle branch blocks' in an ECG graph may be described as left or right. A left bundle branch block may be associated with a heart condition. If the block is in the right side of the heart, right bundle branch block, it is likely to be a variation of normal heart functioning.

Soon I also put that test behind me.

"I will show it to my boss," the assistant said. "We shall do the exercise ECG after he has seen it."

"May I please cast a glance at it?" I asked.

"No problem; I forgot that you are also a doctor."

I was positively surprised at what I saw. Apart from the changes already referred to, there was nothing that pointed to a clinically significant heart condition. The heartbeat was 60 per minute, which was the lowest of what is considered normal.

On her return, she asked me to follow her to the cubicle where the exercise ECG was to take place. Here, too, I shall pause to provide the reader with a short overview of the examination. As the name suggests, it is an ECG test done during exercise. It is capable of detecting heart abnormalities that a resting ECG is incapable of doing. The test can be done with the help of a stationary bicycle or a treadmill. The patient has to walk on a motor-driven treadmill or pedal a stationary bicycle as the case may be. It is used among other things to help find the causes of unexplained chest pain, dizziness, fainting, irregular heartbeat and also to check for a blockage or narrowing of the vessels that supply the heart.

In my case a stationary bicycle was used. Here the patient is required to pedal fast enough to maintain a certain speed. The resistance is then gradually increased in stages, each lasting about three minutes, making it harder to pedal. As one exercises, the ECG and heart rate are recorded continuously. The blood pressure is also measured at regular intervals. The entire test usually takes 15 to 30 minutes to complete. Among other things, the test may be stopped when the patient begins to show symptoms of fatigue, extreme shortness of breath, irregular heartbeat or an extreme rise or fall in blood pressure.

In Germany the law requires that a doctor is present throughout the test. After waiting for about 15 minutes Michael arrived. As is customary in Germany for GPs and hospital doctors, he was dressed all in white—a white pair of trousers, white shirt and long white coat. After exchanging warm greetings we got down to business.

During my student days I used to ride on my bike to lectures. That involved riding a distance of about 10 kilometres. Of late, however, I had almost abandoned the habit of cycling. This was reflected in my performance on the stationary bike. After about seven minutes, the examination was called off, not due to problems related to my heart, but as a result of general fatigue.

Just as I had finished putting on my clothes, Michael turned to me:

"Come along, friend, I want to carry out an ultrasound scan."

Also known as diagnostic sonography, ultrasound scans are images of the internal organs created from sound waves. The images are produced when the sound waves are directed into the body and then reflected back to a scanner that measures them. They can help identify diseased conditions in organs such as the liver, kidneys, the womb, the prostate gland, etc.

As requested, I followed my doctor friend to one of the several examination rooms spread over the two floors of his large modern practice. Moments later I was lying on an examination bed beside a modern ultrasound device, with the top part of my body exposed. One after the other my experienced friend scanned my internal organs—the liver, the bile duct, the pancreas, both kidneys, the abdominal section of the aorta (the largest artery of the body) and the prostate. Next, he placed the device on my neck to check the thyroid gland (a two-lobed endocrine gland located at the base of the neck that secretes chemicals that regulate the rates of metabolism, growth, and development).

Finally he placed the device on both sides of my neck to look out for possible narrowing of the large vessels leading from the heart to the brain.

"Everything is fine, my friend."

"That is good news; very good news."

He was not finished with me, though, not until he had carefully listened to my heart with his stethoscope.

"Any problems?" I inquired after he had returned the device to one of the pockets of his coat.

"None that I can report about, friend!" His words were followed by a short silence broken by the concluding observation of my caring friend. "I really do not think there is any problem with your heart. Still, I will refer you to the cardiologist for the echo."

"Please do that. I want to be 100 per cent certain the problem is not heart related."

"When do you intend returning to the UK?"

"The day after tomorrow."

"I cannot get an appointment at such short notice; you will have to come back another time."

"No problem."

"The blood test results will be ready tomorrow. You can collect them before your departure."

"Okay; see you tomorrow."

"No, I won't be around. I work elsewhere on Thursdays. The surgery will be open though."

I went for the results the next day as planned. A pleasant surprise awaited me when the report was handed to me.

It might well have been that of a healthy 18-year-old!

No sign of inflammation, no anaemia (indeed I had so much blood I would make a good donor), and I had optimal liver, kidney and thyroid functions! The only value that was slightly raised was my sugar level. I put this down to the fact that I ate too late the previous night. The reader will recall that I arrived in Dusseldorf after 10 p.m. We eventually got home around midnight. I knew that was not the right thing to do because of the impending investigations the next day. Since I was hungry, however, I was tempted to eat something. If indeed my sugar level was raised, that should not come as a surprise to me—it should only serve as a warning to me to mind my diet, for I was indeed at risk. My mother passed away as a result of complications related to Type II diabetes, the type of diabetes associated with old age. It is that type of diabetes that can be inherited. Indeed, one of my brothers is plagued with the condition.

As I flew back to the United Kingdom I occupied my mind with my problem and its possible cause. Now that the ECG, both at rest and under exercise, the ultrasound scan of all the major organs as well as the urine and blood had all turned out fine, I felt vindicated in my suspicion that there was no bodily cause for the problem. Still, I was keen to undergo the echo. That would provide definitive clarity in the matter.

-12-

AN ABRUPT ENDING TO A WEEK'S ASSIGNMENT

SEVERAL WEEKS BEFORE the unexpected trip to Germany, my agency had booked me to work from Monday 3rd till Friday 7th October in a prison near Norwich, a city about 200 kilometres to the south-east of Loughborough.

On my return from Germany on Friday 30th September, my prayer to the Lord was to show me favour to enable me to honour the assignment. Having missed the earnings from the previous week, the family coffers could hardly withstand any further loss of income.

As I mentioned earlier, when I work far away from home, I leave home early on the first working day and stay in a bed and breakfast until the last working day. That was the case on this occasion also. I went through the session on Monday without any problems. The same was the case on Tuesday, Wednesday and Thursday. As was the case throughout the week, the session on Friday was due to end around 5 p.m. I would then drive home.

As I had done throughout the week, I came out of the prison around 12:30 p.m. on an hour's break. I used the opportunity to call Rita to let her know everything was fine with me. Shortly after doing that I headed for the staff canteen, which happened to be outside the main prison building.

Just as I sat down to enjoy the meal I had ordered, the pattern of symptoms the reader is now familiar with—hotness of the whole body, a racing heart followed by dizziness—set in.

"One more time!" I said to myself, almost at the point of exasperation. I could barely stay on my seat as the world began to spin before my eyes.

After remaining still for a while, I felt some relief so far as the feeling of dizziness was concerned. Not so the feverish feeling of the body. Feeling uncomfortable, I decided—though reluctantly—to dispose of the meal I had barely touched and seek fresh air.

After sitting outside for a while I felt strong enough to return to the prison. As I went, it became clear to me that there was no way I could work the afternoon session. On reaching the health care unit I headed for the office of the manager.

"I am terribly afraid I have to abandon the afternoon session," I began.

"That cannot be true, doc!" she replied, surprised.

"I am afraid I am experiencing a dizzy spell. They have been recurring of late. I felt fine throughout the week. Unfortunately it has returned!"

"That is really unfortunate. The prisoners have already been collected from their cells!"

"Well, I am very sorry about that. There is little I can do. Even as I speak with you, I do not feel steady on my feet."

Soon I was heading out of the prison, feeling not only hot within myself but also quite dizzy. Would I be able to make the three-hour drive home? As on previous occasions, I prayed to the good Shepherd to shepherd me home. As I drove on, I gave Him thanks for the opportunity to work that week. Having worked four full days and a half, I had earned enough money to keep the family going for the next several days.

Rita, who was expecting me several hours later, was surprised to see me when I pulled up outside our home (I had not informed her about the incident).

"I thought you would be arriving around 9 p.m.!" she exclaimed as I entered the house.

"Well, here I am!"

"What happened?"

"Well, the old problem set in not long after I had spoken to you."

"Once again!"

"Well, there is nothing I can do about it, except to pray. The forces of hell are up against me. I am not scared though—never!"

Over the next two weeks I struggled to work through the few sessions that had been booked for me several weeks earlier.

I could have taken the initiative to look for more work by calling the locum agencies myself. Due to reasons that the reader is already familiar with, I decided not to take that step, at least not until I had done the echo. Michael had in the meantime e-mailed me to inform me he had booked me for the said test for Thursday 3rd November.

-13-

ONE MOMENT 'MR DOCTOR', THE NEXT 'MR PATIENT'!

ON THURSDAY October 20th, almost four weeks to the day of the events of 24th September that the reader is aware of, I returned to work for the first time in the same London prison. I was booked to work from 2.00 to 10 p.m. with an hour's break between 5.00 and 6.00 p.m.

I left home around 10:30 a.m. for the drive to London. As is my custom when driving, I occupied myself listening to gospel music. To inform myself about possible congestions on the road and what was happening in the world, I occasionally tuned in to the radio.

It was on one of such switches from the CD player to the radio that the breaking news about the capture of the late Colonel Gaddafi, then the Libyan leader, was reported by the BBC. Initially the talk was about him having been captured alive. In the course of my drive the same station carried the news of his possible death. Just at the time of my arrival at my destination, the station quoted a high-ranking member of the transitional government confirming his death. Life! How unpredictable it can be—one day alive, the next day gone, I reflected.

My duty on that day involved two sessions. The first session was from 2 to 5 p.m. It involved seeing and reviewing the prescriptions of inmates already in the establishment. The second session was between 6 and 10 p.m. It was devoted to inmates sent to the prison on that day. Inmates arriving in the prison on a particular day could be placed in two categories—those who had been transferred from another prison and those sent there from the courts.

The new inmates are first screened by the nurses. They refer those needing to see the doctor to the doctor's consultation room. One might wonder why they are sent to prison if they need medical attention. The answer is that they are usually not acutely ill. Those who fall into that category at the time of their arrest are usually admitted to hospital.

Those sent to prison are deemed medically fit to be there. The doctor seeing inmates on the day of their arrival in the establishment has the duty of prescribing the medication they were on prior to their arrival. For legal reasons, the medication prescribed by an outside doctor cannot be administered in the prison until they have been re-prescribed by a prison doctor.

A good proportion of individuals sent to prison in the United Kingdom are addicted to various substances—heroin, alcohol, diazepam, etc. It is the duty of the doctor seeing such inmates on their arrival to prescribe substitute medication that will permit them to serve their various sentences without going into withdrawal.

Midway through the first session my body began gradually to experience a sensation of hotness, similar to the one the reader is familiar with.

The particular doctor's room where I was boasted two windows, each of which was larger than the one I referred to earlier. I took a look at them—one was already tilted open, the other was shut. Still feeling very uncomfortable, I opened the second one also.

The nurse who was assisting me had gone to collect the next patient so she did not notice what I had done. It was a chilly autumn evening. Opening the second window had led to an inflow of a stream of chilly wind. Though I could feel the cold on the surface of my body, the inside of my body continued to feel as if on fire!

"It's freezing in here, doc, let's close one of the windows," the nurse suggested after a while.

"I am feeling hot and uncomfortable my dear, please let's keep it open."

"Well, maybe it's me—I put on light clothing today; I need to put on something warmer next time."

If only she would realise the problem was not with the way she had dressed! Instead it lay with me—I was burning in my body, and it was I who needed the cold wind to provide some relief!

I really had to struggle through the session. Though feeling uncomfortable, I was determined to see all the patients booked for attention. Fortunately for me about a third of those on the list failed to turn up, enabling me to finish several minutes ahead of schedule.

The second session was to be held in the doctor's room on the E-wing of the prison, the same room I had used on the Saturday I fell ill at work.

After taking my seat in the new location, I realised I still had about half an hour before the evening session, so I decided to while away my time surfing the internet.

At around 5:45 p.m. a pleasant gentleman aged about 40, a citizen of Nigeria, entered the room.

"Doc, I am assigned to you today."

"That's great; I hope we will have a quiet session."

"Well, you know how unpredictable the session can be. Today a few new arrivals, the next day several of them!"

"Well, let's hope for the best!"

At that juncture he took a look at his watch.

"Doc, are you ready to start?"

"What's the time?"

"5:45."

"Okay, let's get going."

"I will go and fetch the first one."

With that he left the room.

Hardly had he stepped outside than I began suddenly to experience the familiar sensation of hotness to my head and body. As if in conflict with my own body, I said to myself, "Enough of that! Not at the time when I have just sent for the first patient!"

Well, that would turn out to be wishful thinking, for just about that moment I felt, as on previous occasions, as if someone was shaking my heart! Soon my heart began to accelerate! With the onset of the tachycardia came the dizziness. Soon, I felt like collapsing to the floor.

Fortunately, there was an examination bed in the room. Moments later I was lying on it, the whole world spinning before me.

"Physician, heal thyself!" someone might want to point out to me. Mortal man that I am, I felt completely powerless in the situation! Friends, we are nothing. If there is anything worthy to hold on to, it is indeed Almighty God, the immortal one. Indeed, after all the years I have spent studying medicine, yes after all the years I have spent helping others, I was literally knocked out in the twinkling of an eye—in a second!

Not long after I had taken my position on the bed, the nurse arrived with the patient!

"Doc, what are you doing?" he inquired in amazement, seeing me on the bed. "I saw the Health Care Manager heading in this direction. You do not want her to see you sleeping on the job, do you?"

"My friend, call for help. The doctor himself needs help!"

For a moment he stood there flabbergasted, clearly not able to fathom what was happening before his eyes.

"This must be a joke!"

"Seriously, friend, I am feeling unwell, so please call for help."

The Health Care Manager had, in the meantime, reached the area. Since the door was open, she noticed what was going on in the room. Without hesitation she entered the room.

"What is happening, doc?"

"I am feeling very unwell, madam. I am feeling very dizzy; my heart is racing within me!"

The news of the duty doctor who had almost collapsed at work spread like wildfire, for soon several nurses rushed to my aid.

"Get his BP checked!" I heard one say.

"Let's give him oxygen; someone please hurry and fetch the cylinder!" another cried out.

Soon the BP cuff was fastened round my upper arm. Moments later the electronic device displayed the result: BP 95/70, pulse 145/min.

Just then one of them arrived with oxygen. Soon I was privileged to be breathing in the life-saving gas.

Just about that moment the manager turned to me: "Should we call the ambulance, doc?"

Doctors are said to be unwilling patients. I think I am no exception. I really did think I would survive the attack just as I had done on the previous two occasions, without the need to go to hospital.

The setting this time was different, however. Not only was the head of health care a witness to the unfolding drama, but several other individuals—nurses, prison officers as well as a considerable number of prisoners—were also present. I needed to set a good example as a doctor. Besides that, I continued to feel my heart racing within me.

There was no chest discomfort, however, something that would lead me to consider a more serious condition such as a possible heart attack.

"Yes, please go ahead and call the ambulance," I replied after a short while.

I had worked in the prison setting long enough to know that it usually takes more than the average time required in a normal setting for the emergency service to arrive at the prison. Though these services do not have to go through the usual security checks, they usually have to go through a few gates, and each gate remains closed until the vehicle is a few metres away.

At that time of day, it was also likely that the roads were congested. Although they have priority on the road, when streets are jammed with traffic as can sometimes be the case in the British capital, the going can be difficult even for the paramedics.

Happily, it took less than 10 minutes for the paramedics to arrive. After the initial checks, they fastened me onto a special chair and got ready to wheel me to the emergency vehicle parked in a courtyard about 50 metres away. Just before we set out the Health Care Manager turned to me and inquired:

"Doc, could you please provide us with your home telephone so we can call your family to let them know about your whereabouts?"

"That is very kind of you, madam. For the moment, however, I want to keep them in the dark."

"Why?" she inquired, somewhat surprised.

"They live in Loughborough, about 110 miles away. I want to spare them the distress, for now, for after all they cannot visit me in the short term. I will let them know in the course of the evening."

"You have to take your wallet with you, doc," another staff member advised me. "You'll need money for the taxi in case you are discharged."

At that moment it occurred to me that I had left my wallet in my car. Partly as a result of the regular checks at prison gates, and also due to the fact that on one occasion my wallet was stolen by an inmate (the thief dumped it on the corridors of the prison after making away with a twenty-pound note in it), I had made it a point to leave it in my vehicle. (While aware that this practice was not entirely devoid of risks, I considered it the lesser of two evils.) On hearing this, the ambulance crew offered to stop at the parking lot to give me a chance to pick it up. They kept to their promise. Though still feeling very poorly, I managed to walk the approximately 20-metre distance to fetch it.

Soon we were negotiating the fairly congested streets heading for hospital. Though my heart continued to beat fast leading me still to feel dizzy, I was alert and "clinically stable" as the medical experts would put it. Though slightly short of breath, I was able to converse well with the paramedic attending me.

As the ambulance continued on its way to A&E, my thoughts went back to the time I used to work as an emergency doctor in Germany. As I recalled those moments, one particular instance came back strongly to mind. On that occasion, the call reached us to attend to a young man aged about 20 who had turned blue and was not breathing properly. His relatives had discovered him in that condition in his room in their large family home. Soon we were speeding through the streets of the medium-sized town. The fact that the address happened to be relatively close to the hospital and also that it was late in the night, leaving the streets deserted of traffic, allowed us to reach him in no time. He was lying on a mattress in their large living room surrounded by about half a dozen very anxious family members. We began immediately to resuscitate him. As it turned out, it was a case of heroin overdose. As I hurried to inject the appropriate medicine to help revive him, my prayer was that the Lord would help me get him safe and alive to A&E.

Though it was not my fault he found himself in that life-threatening situation, I could only imagine what would happen should the worse happen and he passed away. All of a sudden experts both in the field of medicine and law would become involved in the case. Soon questions as to whether the emergency doctor acted appropriately, whether he could not have done more to avert the situation, would have been raised.

On that occasion, and on all other occasions during my work as a doctor, I was the provider of help. Now I was experiencing a role reversal. Oh, poor humanity! One moment he/she is the doctor treating patients; the next moment, he/she is being rushed to A&E, at the mercy of others.

For the first time in over 28 years I found myself as a patient in a hospital setting. The last time I found myself in that situation was in 1983. In contrast to the journey I was undertaking to hospital along the streets of London, my journey to hospital on an underground train of West Berlin was planned. On that occasion I was admitted to the Oskar Helena Heim, a renowned orthopaedic clinic in the capitalist part of the divided city. Although it may sound strange, on that occasion I was happy to be in hospital. Why would anyone be happy about the prospect of being admitted to a hospital, someone might wonder? The answer is that the admission and routine surgery planned on my left ankle offered a promising prospect of bringing to an end an ailment that had plagued the said ankle since my boyhood days. And that turned out to be the case. Since I underwent the procedure in the first week of February 1983, I have had peace from the 'terror' of the pain that until then had been recurring at regular intervals.

On this my second visit to hospital, more than 28 years on, the circumstances were entirely different. It was not an issue involving an ankle bone. Instead it was a matter of the heart of all organs! Was it a heart muscle disease (what the medical people term cardiomyopathy?) Was it coronary heart disease? Was my dutiful heart on the point of putting an end to its activities and so bringing an end to my stay on planet earth?

-14-
IN ATTENDANCE AT A MINI UNITED NATIONS GATHERING

THE SITUATION that confronted me at Accident and Emergency led me to think I was perhaps attending a mini-gathering of the United Nation rather than visiting the A&E department of a hospital in Europe. It did indeed appear to me as if people of all colours, religions, continents and what-have-you were represented. Be it a patient, a nurse or a doctor, all kinds of God's children were gathered here. I was aware that the United Kingdom, partly as a result of its history, partly as result of the shortage of nurses and doctors, has traditionally recruited overseas medical personnel, in particular from the former colonies. I had the opportunity to see things for myself.

On arrival, the paramedics placed me at one corner of the waiting area. One of them remained with me while the other went to report on my case. Seated just in front of me were two elderly women, both aged about 60. Soon I overheard them conversing in the *Twi* language. What, I wondered, had led the two elderly citizens of my native country to A&E?

"You better concern yourself with what is happening in your own back yard rather than poke your nose over other people's fences to inquire about what is happening in their home," urged a voice within me.

Indeed I needed first to sort out what was happening to me rather than occupy myself with issues relating to others. Surely, there was the need to find out as quickly as possible what was going on in me. Since the investigation in Germany had been fine, the only important part of the investigation that was outstanding was the echocardiography. How

I wished I could bring forward the appointment in Germany to the next day or the day thereafter!

As I sat there pondering on what could be wrong with my heart, I recalled the telephone conversation I had with an acquaintance of mine, a citizen of Ghana resident in London. He had called to request me to explain the term 'cardiomyopathy'. I wanted to know why he wanted to know. To that he replied that a citizen of Ghana resident in the British capital had died suddenly of the condition. The English GP of the dead man had explained the term to them. Partly as a result of the language barrier they had not completely grasped what the medical expert had told them. He wanted me therefore to explain the 'awkward' medical term in the *Twi* language. I did my best to explain the condition in the language requested. Was I myself also plagued with the heart condition with the clumsy name?

This was to be my first experience with the UK medical system as a patient since my arrival from Germany. I have in the meantime heard and read reports concerning long waiting hours at A&Es on the island. I had the opportunity to verify things for myself.

Was it because of the nature of my problem? Was it because the paramedics revealed to them who I was and the circumstances surrounding my case? Whatever the reason, I was attended to reasonably quickly. Indeed, not long after my arrival, I was wheeled into one of the consulting rooms.

Soon I was attended to by a female nurse whose age I estimated to be about 25. As it turned out, she happened to be from Nigeria. After she had introduced herself, she asked me to remove the clothing on the upper part of my body and climb onto the examination bed. Soon she set about fixing the ECG cables on to my body. A look on the monitor of the device told me my pulse was still high—130/min.

After she had printed it, she left the room. She needed to show it to the doctor, she told me.

Not long after she had left, a male nurse of Asian descent, whose age I estimated to be about 30, entered the room. He was there to take blood samples, he announced. A few minutes later he was on his way out of the room, having carried out his task.

-15-

A GHANAIAN PATIENT UNDER THE CARE OF A NIGERIAN DOCTOR IN THE UK!

AFTER WAITING for about 15 minutes, a slender-looking lady in a green outfit—green pair of trousers and a green top—entered the room. She carried a stethoscope over one of her shoulders.

"Good evening, sir. My name is Dr N [full name omitted]," she introduced herself.

"Good evening, madam," I replied. "It is a pleasure meeting you."

"I am the doctor on duty."

"That is great. I hope you can help get to the bottom of my problem."

"I will do my best."

A short silence followed. It was broken by me.

"Are you from Nigeria?" I asked inquisitively.

"Yes, what led you to that conclusion?"

"Your first name. I have some connections to your country. I once taught in Shagamu, in the Ogun state. Beside that I have several Nigerian friends and acquaintances."

"And you—where are you from. Ghana?"

"Your guess is right. A Ghanaian patient being treated by a Nigerian doctor in Europe—welcome to the global village!"

"Well, the world has indeed become a small place."

"A young doctor bubbling with energy and enthusiasm!" I remarked, beginning to enjoy her company. "I am getting old. You notice my black hair is losing the battle with the grey hair."

"What makes you think I am young?"

"Pardon me if that is not the case. I seem to have been deceived by your looks."

"Well, I am not all that young. In any case, can you please give me a brief history of your condition?"

I obliged and gave her a summary.

"So you are booked for the echo in Germany?"

"Yes. I am due to have it on the 3rd of November—that's about two weeks from now. Or can I have it earlier in the UK?"

"I can't guarantee that. Unless, of course, tonight's investigation leads us to think you need one without delay. Now I will leave you alone to rest whilst we await the outcome of the blood test."

She returned a short while later.

"I have requested a chest x-ray," she began. "Will you please follow me as I direct you to the place?"

She directed me to the x-ray department when we stepped outside.

I thought the idea of the x-ray was good. Among other things it might give us a clue as to whether a condition afflicting the heart had led to my symptoms, such as an enlarged heart. I did not have to wait long before I was called into a room where the x-ray was to be done. Soon, I had that behind me too.

In the meantime, I continued to feel stronger and stronger. Feeling my pulse told me the rate at which my heart was beating had reduced to around 90 per minute.

The clock on the wall in the meantime read 10:05 p.m. That was about the time I would normally be ringing my family to bid them goodnight. It then occurred to me that I did not have my mobile phone with me, having left it in my vehicle before entering the prison. (It is strictly forbidden to take a mobile phone into a UK prison; one could be prosecuted if caught with it.)

What was to be done? I talked to Dr N about the matter.

"No problem, doc, you can use our phone," she said, pointing to a phone on the reception desk. Soon I was dialling our number.

At the first attempt no one picked up the phone. I waited a few minutes and redialled. This time Jonathan, our 10-year-old son, picked it up.

"How are you, boy?" I said.

"Fine. The display on the phone is reading 'Private'. That is why I refused to pick it up earlier on."

The young boy was indeed acting upon instructions, having been told not to pick up calls that are not familiar to him.

"Well, it is me, boy."

"Where is your mobile phone, Papa? Why are you not using it?"

"I will tell you later. You call your mother."

"She is in the bathroom."

"Okay, then I will hang up now. Tell her I will call again in a few minutes."

I repeated the call after about 20 minutes. This time his mother was on the line.

"Jonathan is still wondering where your mobile phone is," she remarked after the exchange of greetings.

"It is in my vehicle!"

"Where then is your vehicle?"

"In the prison parking lot."

"Where are *you* then?"

"At the A&E!"

"The A&E!"

"Yes, you heard me right. I was rushed to the A&E of the St George's Hospital. It happens to be the nearest hospital to the prison. My problem returned around 6 p.m. I was rushed here in the ambulance!"

"The ambulance! Is everything alright?"

"No worries, I am now feeling better. I will not spend the night here. I am just waiting for the doctor to discharge me. I will spend the night at the B&B and return home in the morning. I will call if I get out before midnight; otherwise you will hear from me tomorrow."

Rita was silent towards the end of the conversation. I knew her well enough to realise she was shocked to the core. How else should she react when someone who left home in quite good health ends up being rushed to A&E!

Doctors are generally said to be impatient patients. Well, judging from my reaction, you might well place me in that category. After returning from the x-ray department, I began, at short intervals, to glance at my watch.

I wished Dr N would come to discharge me. Finally, at around 11 p.m., she arrived.

"The x-ray is fine," she said. "All the blood values are fine. The only exception is the troponin which is slightly raised. Our protocol requires us, under the circumstances, to repeat the value after three hours. If it turns out to be still high, you may have to spend the night here."

The layman may wish to know that troponin is a value in the blood which can become elevated in response to muscle—in this case heart muscle—damage The damage to the heart muscle in its turn can be due to factors such as heart attack or severe tachycardia (a racing heart).

In my case, I put the elevated troponin value down to a racing heart. Having been beating around 140 times per minute for several minutes instead of 60 per minute as is usually the case with me, it did not come as a surprise to me that the said value was raised.

Eventually we agreed on a compromise—the blood test would be retaken and she would inform me of the result in case it was still raised (indeed, she informed me a few days later that had been the case). In return I signed a disclaimer to the effect that I was leaving the hospital at my own volition.

At around 11:20 p.m. I left the gates of the hospital in a taxi that brought me to the parking lot of the prison.

Finally at around 11:40 p.m. I pulled up at the gates of the B&B. I called home to break the news to Rita.

The manager of the B&B was waiting for me. He was his usual friendly self. Knowing that I would be working till Saturday, I had booked two nights, Thursday and Friday.

"How was work today, doc?"

"Not good, friend, not good."

"What happened?"

"I felt unwell at work."

A short silence followed.

"Now, would you please remind me about your booking terms? Is it too late to cancel tomorrow's booking now? I will stay for one night instead of two."

"I am afraid it is too late," he replied. "It will be difficult to find a replacement at such short notice. So I am afraid you will have to pay for the two nights. I do promise you though that should we, contrary to expectation, find a replacement we shall refund the money during your next stay."

It was a few minutes past midnight when I finally retired to bed.

I woke up early to drive back home, long before the London rush hour traffic could start building up to delay my journey. Throughout that day, Friday, I was fine.

-16-
A DESPERATE ATTEMPT TO APPLY THE BRAKE ON A RACING HEART

I SEEM TO HAVE PASSED ON my passion for football to my little boy Jonathan. Though I used to be actively engaged during my younger years, my passion for the game is now restricted to watching it occasionally on TV. Not so the 10-year-old lad! He plays in a junior side of Loughborough Dynamos Football Club. Saturday morning between 10 and 12 a.m. is their training time.

When I am off duty, I drive him to the training ground about two kilometres from our home; otherwise the duty falls on his mother.

On that Saturday I dropped him at the training ground and returned home to rest for a while. I returned about 15 minutes before the end of the training session to fetch him. Just as I got out of the vehicle, the now familiar pattern of the disease set in! I saw two options—to wait for him or to drive back home and ask his mother to do so. In the end I decided to hang on.

If only the trainer knew what was going on in me! Obviously he did not. Thus instead of ending the session on time, he allowed the kids to play on for almost 10 minutes beyond the scheduled time. At one stage I had wanted to signal Jonathan to desert the game and come along. On second thoughts, I refrained from doing so. I could imagine the consternation in his face had I interrupted his game in that manner.

To my relief, the trainer finally blew his whistle to bring the training to a close. As I drove home, an idea occurred to me to make an attempt at what is known in medical jargon as a symptomatic therapy. As the name suggests, this type of therapy aims at the symptoms of disease, not the cause. As far as the hotness in the head and body was concerned there was not much I could do about it, for the hotness was not due to a rise in bodily temperature that could be treated with relevant medication. Not so the racing heart: in that instance I could resort to a group of medication known as beta blockers to contain it.

This is not the proper forum for a detailed lecture on this group of medication. For our present discussion, it is sufficient for the reader to know that beta blockers work in the body to, among other things, reduce the rate of heartbeat and also the blood pressure. Under normal conditions I would not consider taking them, since my blood pressure is usually low. In view of the events of the last several days, however, I resolved to give them a try. I would not take them regularly; instead, I would take them only when needed. I would balance the need to reduce the heartbeat with the need to maintain an adequate blood pressure.

There are several types of beta blockers in use. In the end I settled on Atenolol. Soon I put words into action and acquired a packet of the said medication. That very evening I had to take some, for, as if to let me know that my affliction was still a force to be reckoned with, the symptoms of the disease returned with a vengeance.

After having a good night's sleep I was greeted on waking up with the now familiar set of symptoms. In my exasperation, I decided to take not half a tablet as on the previous occasion, but instead a whole tablet!

I was aware it could reduce my BP considerably, but the Christian soldier had reached the point of frustration on account of the apparent delay of the Great Redeemer to intervene in the situation.

What I had feared became reality; though the pulse had reduced to 90 for the most part of the day, the medication led to a considerable reduction of my blood pressure. At one stage my BP fell to a level as low as 85/45! For most of the day I was forced to remain in the lying down position, hardly able to balance myself on standing up.

I was booked to work in a prison situated about 120 kilometres to the north of our home the next day, Monday. The assignment was to last until that Friday. I realised that cancelling the session on Monday could lead the agency to pass on the whole week's assignment to someone else. Having lost the income of the last several days, I saw the need to honour the assignment at all costs. If our financial situation at that time was comparable to a patient that has been admitted to a normal ward, failure to earn any income the following week could mean a worsening of the condition of the patient to the point that would warrant a transfer to the intensive care ward!

I began to lift up my eyes to the Hills for help. I pleaded with Heaven to consider in particular our son David who, as I mentioned earlier, has the condition of autism. Karen, our 19-year-old, and perhaps Jonathan too, could understand the need for austerity at home under the present circumstances. As far as David is concerned, however, food must be ready when needed!!

Towards the evening I began to feel a bit better, to the extent that I could take a few steps. The BP had risen to around 90/70; the pulse had settled around 80 per minute.

Despite my condition I was determined to go to work the next day, come what may.

-17-

"GIVE A CLAP OFFERING FOR JESUS!"

WHEN I WOKE UP the next morning I felt miserable, to put it mildly. I measured my BP: 100/65, pulse 100. I wished at that moment I was in regular employment. I would have taken the phone, called my boss and reported sick.

A look at the watch told me it was 6:45 a.m. The session was to begin at 8:30 a.m. It would take me around 90 minutes' drive to get there.

What was to be done? Call my agency to cancel my assignment and risk losing a whole week's income, or head for work, trusting in the protecting arms of the Good Shepherd?

In the end I decided in favour of the latter. Still not quite stable on my feet, I took a deep breath, fetched my doctor's bag as well as the house and car keys and headed outside.

"I am going to pass through the valley of the shadow of death. Please preserve me, Lord," I prayed. Saying that, I turned the house key, opened the door and stepped outside.

As I got into my vehicle, not only did I feel quite dizzy, I also felt hot in my body. I opened the windows of the vehicle halfway to let in the cold breeze of the autumn morning. The time, meanwhile, was 6:55 a.m.

"The Lord is my shepherd, I shall not want!" I whispered into the air and inserted the ignition key.

"Lord, you know how much I need this money to feed the family, so take me there and back!" With that I turned the key. Moments later I was on my way.

As I drove on, I felt increasingly better. Finally after driving for about an hour and a half, I reached my destination. Apart from a few bursts of dizzy spells I managed to get through the day's assignment without much difficulty.

When I reached home in the evening the first thing I said to my family was: "Come on everyone, give a clap offering to Jesus!"

The next day, Tuesday, the morning session went without any problem. Not so the afternoon session. Just as I was about halfway through the four-hour session, my heart began to race again; soon I began to feel dizzy. I felt my pulse: it had risen to 120. Just then it occurred to me that I had left in the vehicle the medication that I had decided to carry on me always.

Though without the medication, I knew there was Someone more powerful than medication I could appeal to for help. And He did help—both directly and indirectly. About 10 minutes after it all began, my pulse went down to 90.

Usually the inmates book the doctor's appointment several days ahead. Often, the problem that caused them to make the appointment with the doctor resolves itself before their turn comes. Some inmates who book sessions also fail to turn up for other reasons. In the end just about half of those on my list for the day turned up, enabling me to end the day almost an hour ahead of schedule. Not long after the last patient left I got the green light to leave for home.

I went through Wednesday without much difficulty. On returning home, I decided to book a bed and breakfast where I would stay after work on Thursday.

I was fine during work on Thursday. On the way to the B&B, I stopped by a supermarket to purchase some food for the evening. Whilst there, my eyes caught sight of an electronic BP machine for sale. Since my device had broken down the previous day, I took advantage of the opportunity to replace it.

Shortly after arriving in my hotel room, my heart began again to accelerate. With the help of the newly acquired machine I checked my values: BP 105/80mmHg, pulse 145/min. In the end I had to resort to the medication already familiar to the reader.

The next day, Friday, I completed my session without any incident.

"Give a clap offering for Jesus!" I urged everyone on reaching home in the evening.

The Mighty Hands of the Lord of Host had seen me through the most difficult working week of my life.

-18-
NEAR SUFFOCATION DEEP UNDER THE SEA BED

ON WEDNESDAY 2nd November, I set out on my second trip to Germany. The echocardiography was scheduled for 11:30 a.m. the next day. This time I opted to drive rather than fly. Several factors led me to my decision. I was accompanied by Karen who had an important appointment in Dusseldorf. It was more economical for us to travel in the family car than to fly or go by train. Besides that, we wanted to do some shopping in Germany which could be transported more conveniently in a car than in the plane or train.

For the sake of those not conversant with the geographical location of the British Isles in relation to the rest of Europe, I shall provide a quick overview.

The United Kingdom is an island lying along the western fringes of mainland Europe. In former times, the only means of reaching the United Kingdom, or the British Isles, from mainland Europe was either by means of sea or air.

In 1988 work began to construct a tunnel deep beneath the English Channel at the Strait of Dover to create a rail link between the United Kingdom and France. The Channel Tunnel was officially opened on 6th May 1994.

The Channel Tunnel, or Eurotunnel as it is also known, is 50.5 kilometres (31.4 miles) long. At its lowest point, it is said to be 75 metres (250ft) deep. The tunnel carries high-speed Eurostar passenger trains as well as Eurotunnel Shuttle roll-on/roll-off vehicle transport trains.

Usually the vehicles are driven by their owners to Folkestone in England and Calais in France as the case may be. The vehicles are then driven and parked in the trains. Passengers are required to remain in their vehicles throughout the crossing, which usually takes around 40 minutes.

I first used the channel crossing in December 1999. That was when I drove with my family from Germany to visit my brother, Ransford, in London. Since then I have used it on several occasions.

I decided on this occasion also to use it as a means of crossing to mainland Europe. I took my medication as well as my BP machine along. Just before the crossing, I checked my BP—it was fine. Hardly had the train set in motion, however, than I began, all of a sudden, to feel the feverish hotness descending on me again! Soon my heart began to race within my chest.

"Not, here, not deep under the ocean bed!" I said to myself. I took a look at the passenger seat. Karen was deeply absorbed in reading a book. Not only that, I could also hear music issuing from the earphone of her iPhone! I wondered what she was enjoying more, the music or the book? I resolved not to disturb her but instead "fight my own fight".

As a first step I took hold of my small travelling bag on the back seat, unzipped it and pulled out the electronic BP machine and set out to check my BP: 110/70, pulse 112 beats per minute. We were in the meantime about five minutes into the journey.

At that moment I decided to take half of the tablet. I had indeed not taken any since the previous evening. I waited a few minutes for an improvement in my condition; no, there was none. I began instead to feel really bad. My fellow traveller was still absorbed in what she was doing.

After a short while I repeated the BP check. 100/70; pulse 145/min. In the meantime I began to feel a shortness of breath. Was I going to collapse deep, deep under the waters of the English Channel?

At that juncture I decided to take more of the medication—this time a whole tablet instead of half a tablet.

After about five minutes, I checked the BP again: BP 90/50; pulse 118. We had in the meantime less than 10 minutes to travel.

I continued, as I had all along, to call on the name of the Lord. "In the Name of Jesus, in the Name of Jesus, in the Name of Jesus...," I kept repeating.

After about 35 minutes, which felt like an eternity to me, the train emerged out of the deep. It still had about five minutes to roll to its station at Calais. Finally it pulled to a halt. The gates were rolled open.

Before long the vehicles parked in it were set in motion by their drivers.

From my previous travels on the route, I was aware there was a service station about a kilometre from the tunnel station. I resolved to stop there and assess my condition before deciding on whether to embark immediately on the 400-kilometre drive to our final destination, or rest awhile before doing so.

Even before I could make my intentions known to her, Karen took a look at me and said: "Let's stop at the next available service station. I need to go to the toilet."

"No worries. I have already made up my mind to stop there to check my blood pressure." BP 90/65, pulse 90/min, was the reading I got.

After standing in the open for about five minutes to enjoy the fresh air, I felt strong enough to continue the journey.

Soon I was behind the wheel. Not long thereafter we were on the highway of France and heading towards Germany. For those not conversant with the geography of the area we travelled, our route passed through the north of France, Belgium and Holland. Dusseldorf lies about 40-kilometres away from the Dutch border.

Frightened by the experience I had had as I went through the Channel Tunnel, I decided to avoid the tunnel on the return journey. If something bad was going to happen to me, then I preferred it to happen in the open rather than deep below the surface of the earth. Initially, my plan was to return by air. I would leave the vehicle in the care of our host and arrange for it to be returned to the United Kingdom at a later date.

As we drove along, however, it occurred to me that one could cross to the United Kingdom by means of the ferry. I could experience seasickness on the journey, but I considered that the lesser of two evils in comparison with the experience just narrated.

The almost four-hour journey to Dusseldorf was uneventful.

Kofi, who had played host to me a few weeks before, was his kind self and welcomed us with open arms into his home.

I decided to put my plans concerning the return journey into action. Consequently I instructed Karen to go online and book the ferry. I thought she would make use of the laptop to do so. However, welcome to the age of the iPhone, smartphone, iPad, and what-have-you! On hearing the instructions, she got hold of her mobile phone.

Shortly thereafter she requested my credit card details. Moments later it was done! For a fee of £39 she had booked a ferry that would head for the United Kingdom at about the same time as the shuttle train we had booked.

-19-
HEART DISSECTION WITH HIGH-TECH

F　**INALLY,** the day for the decisive examination arrived. My first point of call was Michael's practice. Following the bursts of dizzy spells since my first visit, we had decided on a 24-hour ECG investigation. I went there to get the device fitted. For those not familiar with it, here is a brief explanation.

The 24-hour ECG equipment, also known as a Holter monitor or ambulatory electrocardiography device, is a piece of equipment about the size of a Walkman that continuously records heart activity. The box-like device is usually worn at the waist and is attached via leads to three or four recording stickers (ECG electrodes) on the chest over a period of between 24 and 48 hours.

From Michael's practice, I headed for the heart specialist, arriving there several minutes ahead of schedule. About half a dozen patients were already in the waiting room when I got there. After waiting for about 20 minutes, it was finally my turn.

First my BP was taken by the nurse. It was quite low, something that made the examiner wonder. After I revealed the medication I had taken the previous evening, she asked me to remove the clothes from the upper part of my body. Once again my ECG at rest was recorded.

Shortly thereafter I was asked to mount the stationery bicycle and get ready for another exercise ECG. As on the previous occasion with Michael, no sign of ischemia—insufficient supply of blood to my heart muscles—was noted.

Finally the heart specialist, whose age I thought to be around 45 years, started to carry out the echo. I felt tense. Would he discover any sign of significant cardiac disease—heart enlargement, heart muscle weakness, significant valve problems, signs of coronary heart disease?

At this stage I was prepared for anything. As I mentioned earlier, I regarded my good health as a privilege, not a right. My heart after all had been in action for more than half a century.

A textbook of medicine tells us the resting heart usually beats between 60 and 80 times per minute. Even taking the lower rate of 60 beats per minute, I worked out that my heart has been beating around 60x60x24x365 times annually. Even if, according to my current passport, I am 50 years old (mind you, no one issued me with a birth certificate at birth, a fact that has led my date of birth to undergo several alterations with time), that will imply that my heart has been beating 60x60x24x365x50 since I arrived on planet earth, not to mention its activities during the time I rested in my mother's womb! Should it come as a surprise to me if the examination discovered that my faithful friend had begun to show signs of wear and tear?

In the light of the above, I was surprised, albeit pleasantly, when I first saw the pumping action of my best friend on the monitor. Though as a generalist I do not claim to be an expert in the interpretation of such images, I could nevertheless discern through viewing its pumping activity on the monitor that my close companion, yes the mate who has been working around the clock to sustain me, was imbued with a great deal of vitality.

Still, I had to turn to the specialist for whom the heart is, as it were, the source of his daily bread, for his expert assessment.

"Good pumping activity, good blood supply to the muscles, no sign of heart enlargement, a great heart for a person of your age," he pronounced, and continued, "The only problem I can identify lies with the mitral valve. There seems to be a small problem with it. As you can see"—here he pointed to it—"it is not closing as optimally as it should." (I shall spare the reader the details in this regard.) "You know as well as myself that cannot account for your tachycardia," he concluded.

"So what do you think is the problem with my heart?"

"I do not know, friend, I do not know. I can only speculate. It may well be caused by excitations originating from centres outside the sinoatrial node." (The sinoatrial node is the impulse-generating area of the heart—the pacemaker.) "Should the condition persist we could attempt an electrophysiological ablation," he said. (Again, I shall spare the layman the details.)

Like many doctors he did not want to create the impression he was helpless regarding the case before him. I thanked him heartily for his help.

-20-
EMBOLDENED FOR BATTLE

AS I STEPPED OUT of the building and made for my car parked about 500 metres away, I was convinced beyond any doubt that the problem I was plagued with was not a medical problem in the conventional sense. The outcome of the echo had once and for all brought me clarity: I was indeed under demonic attack—under attack from the principalities and powers of darkness.

As I approached my vehicle, I sensed an extraordinary burst of energy descending on me. I had a feeling as if I was David on his way to confront Goliath! Indeed, as far as I was concerned the battle lines were drawn: on the one side Satan with his host of demons; and on the other side myself shielded by the Holy Spirit of the Ancient of Days.

"Look here, demons, I will not allow myself to be intimidated, no, never! In the Name of Jesus of Nazareth, depart from me and make for Hell, where you belong!" I shouted into the air. Someone seeing me may well have considered me crazy! But I was not.

The sister who led me to Christ once told me that Satan does not understand diplomatic language. According to her, the child of God needs to confront him aggressively! That was exactly what I was doing on the streets of Dusseldorf as I headed for my vehicle.

I really do not remember the last time I felt so emboldened in my Christian walk. Like Elijah, I was prepared to confront the prophets of Baal. Like Daniel in the lion's den, I trusted the Lord to send his angels to shut the mouths of the Devil. Like Shadrach, Meshach and Abednego, I trusted the angels of the living God to rescue me from the burning furnace of demonic machinations. Yes, I was prepared in the Name of Jesus to fight back!

From then on I decided not to do anything that would create the impression in the command centre of the Enemy that I was scared or panicky! No, I would not be frightened, or scared or coerced by the antics of the principalities and powers of darkness. To that end I decided to abandon the idea of avoiding travel through the Eurotunnel. As I mentioned earlier, I had on several occasions used it as means of crossing the English Channel. In the same way I had relied on the Lord to preserve me on such occasions before, I trusted Him now to do the same on this occasion.

I began to challenge the forces against me to meet me not at the entrance but instead midway through the journey, very deep under the surface of the earth for battle! They could face me with all the forces they could muster! Shielded by the bloodstained Cross of Calvary, I was confident of victory.

When I got back to Kofi's house I made my plans known to Karen.

"Are we really returning by way of the Eurotunnel?"

"Yes indeed; you heard me right!"

"What made you to change your mind?"

"The doctor did not find anything wrong with my heart. So I do not expect anything to happen during the crossing."

"Should I attempt to claim a refund from the ferry booking?"

"I do not know their terms; you bought the ticket. You check their terms and apply for a refund if applicable."

In the end she gave up trying. It was not very important to me, however. I would after all have forfeited the money paid for the return journey on the Eurotunnel had we gone ahead and travelled by ferry.

We left Dusseldorf the next day as scheduled to drive back to the United Kingdom. Earlier in the morning, I returned the 24-hour ECG device to Michael. He asked me to give him time to interpret and evaluate it. He would e-mail the result to me. As I had expected, the recording of my heart activity over the 24-hour period turned out to be fine.

No, I was no longer afraid! No weapons formed against me would prosper, and I was aware of that. Why indeed should I fear when I have the Lord of hosts for refuge?

As we set out on the return journey to the United Kingdom, I felt emboldened, yes *very* emboldened! I challenged the demons to meet in their thousands, their tens of thousands at the entrance to the Eurotunnel! Like Elijah who confronted the 490 prophets of Baal on Mount Carmen and overcame them, I was also prepared, in the Mighty Name of the Lord of Hosts, to confront the demons, not in my strength but in the strength and might of mighty Jesus. Going into battle in the Mighty Name of Jesus, defeat was not an issue.

After driving for about four hours, we got safely to Calais. After going through the usual security and immigration checks, I drove my vehicle into a waiting Eurotunnel shuttle train. I recalled to mind the assurance of the Lord's superior power of protection:

No weapon that is formed against you will prosper; and every tongue that accuses you in judgment you will condemn. This is the heritage of the servants of the LORD, and their vindication is from Me, declares the LORD. (Isaiah 54:17. New American Standard Bible.)

Prior to departure, I checked my BP. It was fine: 105/70, pulse 66/min. Not long after our arrival, the train set in motion. I began to recite Psalm 23, repeating in particular verse 4:

Yea, though I walk through the valley of the shadow of death, I will fear no evil: for thou art with me; thy rod and thy staff they comfort me.

To uplift my faith further, I played inspiring gospel music. The seconds quickly turned into minutes: 5, 10, 15. I felt fine; no feeling of hotness, no racing of the heart, no shortness of breath. I felt and counted my pulse: 72/min.

About half an hour into the journey I took a look through the window—we had emerged from the tunnel, for I could see street lights in the distance. After travelling a few more minutes the train finally pulled to a halt.

The three-hour drive to Loughborough was uneventful.

-21-

TO GOD BE THE GLORY

ON MY RETURN from Germany, my first session at the London prison the reader is already familiar with was scheduled for Monday 7th November. A few days prior to that date I received an e-mail from my agency to inform me the prison had requested a doctor's note to the effect that I was fit for work. Until that was done, I could not resume work there. I could understand their concern. Having experienced my problem on two occasions they had chosen to tread with caution.

I contacted Michael on the matter.

"No problem," was his reply.

"Will you be happy to do it in English to spare me the need to have it translated?"

"I will try—in the best English I can muster," was his reply.

Not long thereafter he e-mailed the note as promised. All was thus set for my first duty since my unscheduled visit to A&E.

"Are you all right, doc?" the first nurse who saw me on my return inquired.

"I am up and going, my dear, by His grace!" I replied, pointing above.

"Doc, you are back!" the healthcare assistant, who had been my assistant on that fateful day, exclaimed on seeing me.

"Yes indeed. I have been healed by the Mighty Hand of the Lord!"

"Doc, I heard you were unwell," another staff member began on seeing me.

"Yes, I had to be rushed to the A&E."

"That is the last thing one would expect to occur to a duty doctor!"
"Well, that is precisely what happened!"
"Glad to see you again. I must say you look even more refreshed."
"All glory be to the Lord Jesus," I replied.

-22-
VICTORY IN THE CROSS OF CALVARY

IN MY BOOK *Doctor Jesus: the Doctor Who Knows No Bounds,* I stress that conventional medicine and prayer can work hand-in-hand in the treatment of disease.

Unquestionably, whether we pray for the healing of whatever ailment that we face—high blood pressure, diabetes, common infections, etc.—it is my conviction that we can also resort to the insight gained over the years in medical science in the treatment of diseases. It was based on that thinking that I decided to take the beta blockers even as I prayed for healing for my condition.

There are some instances though when medical science comes to the end of its wits in the battle against disease. I recognised such an instance the moment the tests, in particular the echo, failed to pinpoint the cause of my problem. That fact, combined with the mysterious nature of the symptoms, led me to believe firmly that I was subject to attack by principalities, powers and spiritual wickedness in high places, as stated in Ephesians 6:12.

Some will discount my claims for lack of scientific evidence. As I mentioned at the beginning of my discourse, there are those who hold tenaciously to the conviction that anything that is not scientifically proved should not be believed. Demanding scientific proof in an area involving the spiritual sphere of our existence is, in my opinion, tantamount to asking a baby who has not yet gained the ability to speak to give evidence in a court of law concerning a crime he/she has witnessed.

Realising that there was nothing wrong with my body that could explain the symptoms I had been experiencing, I decided to gear myself for the spiritual warfare by way of prayer and meditation on the word of God. Armed with the bloodstained banner of the Cross of Calvary, I geared myself for any future onslaughts of the Devil.

Previously I had been taking the beta blockers on quite a regular basis. I decided to stop that habit. Instead I would resort to it as a very last resort. During the first week of November, on two occasions, I took a tablet to contain brief episodes of tachycardia.

At the time of writing these lines, at the end of December 2011, I have never again had the need to take the said medication. Indeed, I have been free from any attacks of the mysterious disease.

Throughout November and December I have been able to honour every session that I was booked for. The realisation of the financial difficulties that my inability to work over the period mentioned would have brought to me and my family has given me reason to express my gratitude to the Lord of Heaven whenever I reflect on the matter.

-23-

THE BATTLE WAGES ON FOR THE CHRISTIAN SOLDIER

In the world ye shall have tribulation: but be of good cheer, I have overcome the world.
John 16:33b

IT IS NOT FOR NOUGHT that the Christian is compared to a soldier. Indeed, the Christian is a soldier engaged in spiritual warfare. We do not have to provoke the enemy to have an attack launched against us. We may, in order not to provoke him, decide to make a detour around his dwelling. Yes, even if we decide to alter our paths after spotting him kilometres away so as not to incite him, the great Deceiver will nevertheless not be impressed and still carry out his plots aimed at eradicating us. So tribulations we are bound to face, fellow soldier of the Cross, so long as we have breath.

One child of God aptly wrote:

> Since we are not in paradise, but in the wilderness, we must look for one trouble after another. As a bear came to David after a lion, and a giant after a bear, and a king after a giant, and Philistines after a king, so, when believers have fought with poverty, they shall fight with

envy; when they have fought with envy, they shall fight with infamy; when they have fought with infamy, they shall fight with sickness; they shall be like a labourer who is never out of work.

Harry Smith

We should indeed discard the notion that when we are in the Lord all will be rosy. The likely reality is that we shall face trials, indeed one after the other. Our consolation in trouble and affliction, however, is that our Lord has overcome the world and, yes, this means that we are fighting on the side of a winning army.

EPILOGUE

WE ARE NOT QUITTERS

AT THE TIME OF WRITING the revised and abridged edition of my account in February 2019, seven years have elapsed since I placed the final full stop on my original account.

I have enjoyed excellent health since then. Indeed over the period, I have not missed a single day of work by reason of ill health.

As I said in the introduction, my finances and business have been under attack, nevertheless. But what is material and financial loss in comparison to good health? Did I bring anything along to this world? Can I take anything along with me when the command reaches me to quite this present life?

Indeed, as long as I am enjoying good health, I don't care a dime what damage the enemy chooses to inflict on my material possessions. I am assured the ability, yes, the willingness of the Divine to replenish, indeed to restore any loss in His own time. To this end, I take comfort in the following scripture passage:

> *And I will restore to you the years that the locust hath eaten, the cankerworm, and the caterpillar, and the palmerworm, my great army which I sent among you. And ye shall eat in plenty, and be satisfied, and praise the name of the* L*ORD* *your God, that hath dealt wondrously with you: and my people shall never be ashamed.*
>
> Joel 2: 25-26 (KJV)

May the name of the Lord be praised and glorified. Amen!

www.ingramcontent.com/pod-product-compliance
Lightning Source LLC
Chambersburg PA
CBHW071709040426
42446CB00011B/1977